The Day
We Gave Up Health

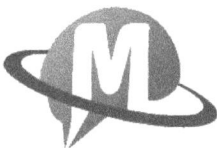

THE MINDTECH
INSTITUTE

www.themindtechinstitiute.com

www.mti.edu.au

©

<u>Copyrights</u>

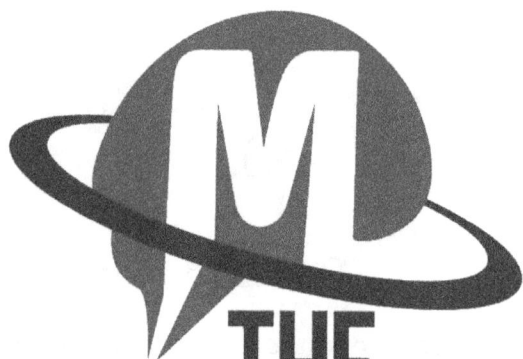

THE
MINDTECH
INSTITUTE

www.themindtechinstitiute.com

www.mti.edu.au

The Day We Gave Up Health

By

Adam Musselli

"A mind is like a parachute. It doesn't work if it is not open."- Frank Zappa.

Dear Reader,

I truly urge you to read this book by putting on your spectacle rather than your skeptical. Read this book with an open mind and see the problems which we're facing rather than ridiculing it or hoping it will disappear by just ignoring it.

People usually put their heads in the sand, just as an ostrich does, for three reasons. The first one is "fear", the second one is "shame" and the third one is "ignoring their existence". The truth sometimes can be frightening, and it might hurt for a while but certainly there's more suffering when we put our heads in the sand for any of the stated reasons.

"Ignorance is not a bliss nor it will ever be and knowledge is not power until it's applied"- Adam Musselli.

"Nothing in life is to be feared, it is only to be understood. Now is the time to understand more, so that we may fear less."

- Marie Curie

"In order to understand something you first need to liberate yourself from it."

- Adam Musselli

INTRODUCTION

At no point in history have humans been so overweight and obese as we are today. The foods we eat and the lifestyles we follow are causing us diseases, illnesses and many other health issues. The very food that is supposed to keep us alive is now leading us on different paths. According to the Centers for Disease Control (CDC), "More than one-third (36.5% or 79.6 million) of American adults are <u>obese</u>". That's right "<u>obese</u>" NOT overweight! Also, according to the Journal of American Medicine (JAMA), in 2008 "The estimated annual medical cost of obesity in the U.S. was $147 billion USD; the medical costs for people who are obese were $1,429 USD higher than those of normal weight". And that's only in the U.S and in 2008. However, the current global figures now are staggering - as you will find out later in this book what is really happening in the U.S, Australia, Europe, Asia, the Middle East and the world!

How in the world did we get so fat in such a short time? Obesity has reached beyond borderlines and it's still rising rapidly. It is noticeable in children, adults and some animals everywhere in the world. Did everyone just get lazy, or acquired food addictions in the past few decades? Or has obesity become an epidemic caused by coincidence? Are we in a new phase of evolution with a new genre of gastronomical habits and foods are so foreign to our bodies causing many generations to suffer in order to become some other evolved species? A new breed of genetic modified and mutated species, or maybe we won't be able to make it this time! Many questions are asked in this book while challenging many organizations and institutions which caused this book to be self-published. This book aims to provide you with honest answers and facts based on high ranked individuals and organizations in the field of medicine, health, politics and research.

What led me to research and write this book is my fascination with the global overweight and obesity phenomena, as well as other related diseases which we are all a part of whether directly or indirectly. It is also the devastating health and economic bill which we're all constantly paying, a member of our families or a member of someone else' family. Indeed, it's a major problem and not many seem to care or at least do something about it.

"The world is a dangerous place to live, not because of the people who are evil, but because of the people who don't do anything about it."- Albert Einstein.

I also wanted to spread this message in a very simple language that makes every person from all walks of life to be able to understand it and share it with others. I believe there are lots of good books on similar subjects also written by doctors and PhDs, but unfortunately, many of them are not easy to read. My goal is to present the facts in a simple way, away from fruitless jargons, and to provide simple and effective answers so that we're all benefitting. The aim of this message is to educate the world about what we're eating and drinking, what is causing illnesses, diseases, deaths and giving simple suggestions to prevent further tragedies.

Many valid points will be covered in this book, such as the what is the so-called 'food' we're eating, how it's affecting us mentally and physically, who's feeding us, the diseases caused by the foods especially diabetes, cancers and other illnesses, and the battles of those who are fighting to lose weight or save their lives. You'll also discover how we've been deceived by the media, other organizations and industries -those we put our trust in their hands and they betrayed us for economic and other personal gains. We will also look at how the media, advertisements and different marketing techniques and campaigns are being used to subliminally direct the masses to various agendas.

You'll learn about why we are getting fatter, GMO foods, fast and processed foods, today's meat, sugar, plastic, fluoride and their effects on our physical and mental health as well as the environment.

Allow me now to show you what I see, to view this world before your eyes with different lenses, a unique spectrum that shows a different reality that may save your life and possibly the world.

Why should I care?!

"First they came for the Socialists, and I did not speak out—

Because I was not a Socialist.

Then they came for the Trade Unionists, and I did not speak out—

Because I was not a Trade Unionist.

Then they came for the Jews, and I did not speak out—

Because I was not a Jew.

Then they came for me—

and there was no one left to speak for me."

- Martin Niemöller (1892–1984)

DISCLAIMER

Raising global awareness is my ultimate goal and I wish that you all enjoy a happy and healthy life.

I would like to apologize in advanced to you my beloved readers if you feel offended in any way while reading this book because that is not what I intended to do. However, the price of the truth is to be able to handle it. I'm not a medical doctor, nutritional doctor nor giving medical advices. This book is fully written based on extensive research in the format of "according to and based on" to deliver to you honest and real facts, not only the opinion of the author.

This book does not provide medical advice, professional diagnosis, opinion, treatment or services to you or to any other individual. This book provides general information for awareness purposes only. The information and suggestions which are provided in this book, are not a substitute for medical or professional care, and you should not use the information and suggestions in place of a medical advice or opinion. Please consult advice from your doctor, physician or other healthcare providers.

You may also notice some points in this book are repeated multiple times. This was done purposely, NOT for the purpose of enforcing an idea – as in "repetition" to make you believe it as the mainstream media does, but to compound the point and present it to you from different approaches.

Lastly, I'm not preaching, advocating or advertising to be vegetarian or vegan. I don't hold a stock on the organic market and I am not trying to spread a conspiracy for personal profit. I'm only providing facts and evidence about issues you might not be aware of. I'm also not preaching or marketing any organization, institution, religion or religious implications even when I use references from religious and other sources. I'm only addressing the subject from all viewpoints such as social, scientific, philosophical, theological, political, spiritual and more. I tried as much as I could not to mention any brands, markets, junk foods and fast food brands to avoid reverse psychology and unintentional advertising and marketing.

The decision is yours!

Adam Musselli

"In times of universal deceit, telling the truth is a revolutionary act."

- George Orwell

"It is not a disgrace to be deceived, but certainly it is to stay in deception."

- Adam Musselli

Contents

"Education is the most powerful weapon which you can use to change the world."

- Nelson Mandela

"Ignorance is not a bliss nor it will ever be, and knowledge is not a great power until it's applied."

- Adam Musselli

Chapter 1
The Evolution of Food

Food and nutrients are fundamental elements in our lives, today our eating habits go further than our simple and necessary nutritional needs. Obesity has become a massive global threat in the developed and developing countries.

However, in order to understand how food addictions, obesity and other related illnesses such as high blood pressure, cancer, sleep apnea, heart diseases, liver diseases, gred (acid reflux), diabetes and many other illnesses related to food and lifestyle, we need to understand first how we got to this point of health adversity. And also understanding the missing link which might balance out the scale again in our favor. Moreover, let's briefly see what has changed in our food chain and how our food has evolved since records began.

Researchers now believe that the sudden rise in obesity in the world is due to a rapid shift in the way we eat. Our food and diet have changed dramatically but our physiology has not. The food or the diet we have now is not matching our physiology, and our physiology doesn't seem to be designed to change or evolve to match such food or diet - and the result is devastating, as we will see in later chapters.

Let's begin by going back in time to the Paleolithic Era around 10,000 years ago. As history and science show, people were nomads, lived by hunting and picking wild fruits and vegetables. According to the University of Utah in 2013 - A Grassy Trend in Human Ancestors' Diets Research, the research indicated that our ancestors' diet was basically made up of protein, fats, fewer carbohydrates with low Glycemic content, high fiber content such as whole grains, leafy vegetables and surely less salt (sodium) if any. And thus, the "Paleo Diet" derives from the diet of the Paleolithic Era.

Our ancestors, during the Paleolithic Era, consumed a large amount of food to provide them with energy, not only because they struggled with the enormous physical demands to hunt, but also because of the living conditions were much more challenging than today and mostly due to the unpredictable weather conditions which forced them to always be on the move from one place to another.

During the latter part of the Stone Age, as our ancestors became more and more inactive, their eating habits suffered the first of the many dramatic changes. Animal breeding allowed them to continue to have meat for consuming (although, not exactly the same quality of meat we have today) while the development of agriculture let them plant their own food and produce cereals such as wheat, rye and barley, and later on pulses such as lentils and peas etc., and lastly, vegetables and fruits.

Since the very beginning, people have lived in harmony with nature. They ate when they needed to eat, hunted when they needed to hunt and didn't consume from nature more than what they needed to, just enough to survive. Obesity and overweight were not common phenomena then until something happened to us in the latter part of the last century.

Several factors drove the situation to escalate, and the major one, it was "ignorance and greed". The "ignorance" of people and the lack of knowledge of what they were eating, what the food contained, and if there were any risks in that food. Also, the "greed" part has the two parties to blame - the people and the food industries. The people's greed is when they started to "live to eat" rather than to "eat to live".

On the other hand, the industry greed is when they started to "extra feed for extra greed".

Furthermore, it was common for people at the time to save small portions of foods for later days. However, since the food industry flooded the market shelves with cheap foods - that caused the human brain to become over-excited and confused. Consequently, such excitement and confusion, caused people to lose track of what and when to eat. And soon later, people started to develop the habit of a "greedy stomach". In addition, the food industries were and still aware of that fact, and they became so irresponsible with their choice of ingredients for easier/cheap process and production, which led them to their greed of faster food production at its cheapest form. The result was a nightmare on our health and the environment.

That was only the history in a nutshell "yesterday leading to now". More details will be further explained later about other specific factors which oversized the world and sickened it.

Obese World

In 2013, the Australian Authoritative Information and Statistics to promote better health and Wellbeing (AIHW), stated, 3 in 5 Australian's are overweight or obese. In 2013, according to the British National Health Service (Public Health England), 62% of adults were overweight in 2012 and 1 in 4 are obese. In the USA, the Centers for Disease Control and Prevention (CDC), stated, more 70.7% of adults age 20 years and over are overweight in 2013 - 2014.

You must be wondering about the statistics on the world scale! Here's your answer. According to the Worldwatch Institute, nearly two billion people worldwide now are overweight and there is a 25 percent increase since 2002. Recently, the American Medical Association voted to classify obesity as a disease, but the question is how strange and quickly that rapid weight-gain happened in just four decades. It is certainly a new kind of epidemic!

Almost a quarter of the world population is battling to lose weight through dieting, exercise and other methods. Certainly, we didn't just wake up one day and found ourselves obese! The honest fact is, we did become lazier and greedy. However, it's not entirely our fault, the companies which are producing our foods have changed the nature of the foods we eat in the last four decades, and that have played a big role in changing our size and the decline of our health. Some people don't even look overweight while their fat is hiding internally, which can be seen on an MRI machine. Although, it's not only about the shape or how we look. It is also about what follows, such as illnesses, cancers, diseases and sometimes death.

Genetically, we haven't changed but our environment and our easy access to cheap and unhealthy food are what has changed. It also became a lot easier and more accessibility to foods compared to 10,000 years ago when we used to be hunters and gatherers. Let us also not forget the media and the food industry that is flooding the market every day with different and new kinds of foods for no other reason but to consume more and more. It's so easy to trick our minds to accept such comfort, and now all this amount of delicious food with various mind-numbing colors sitting on the shelves at the supermarkets waiting for our purchase.

Another reason, we have it all easy and accessible now to get food. You don't need to get out of your car to pick up your food or to go buying fresh foods and vegetables to cut, prepare and cook. All you do now is drive through at any 24/7 fast food restaurant. You don't even have to leave your house if you don't want to, especially if you're watching your favorite TV show. All you need is to pick up your cell phone and order a pizza. And you can also order online or through a phone application if you're too tired to pick up the phone and work your holy fingers to dial the number and talk! We're certainly eating too much, with a minimal level of activity to burn whatever we're eating. But also, it is time to wake up now and acknowledge this fact - the food industry itself is a profit-driven industry, and that's the reason they are putting cheap food on your plate so you can eat more and consume more. This strategy will result in more profit to the food industry. In other words, they wouldn't exist without us!

"What an extraordinary achievement for a civilization: to have developed the one diet that reliably makes its people sick!"

- Michael Pollan

"With evolution, things are always changing, so I sort of think: Should we all be growing three heads?"

- Karl Pilkington

"Always trust someone who is seeking the truth …never trust someone who found it."

- Jordan Maxwell

"There are lots of half –truths around. Watch out if you got the wrong half."

- Adam Musselli

Chapter 2
Who is Feeding Us?

If we ask the general public, who's feeding us? The answer will be the "farmers"! This answer will lead us to a more specific question, which is "who's feeding the farmers"?! Since the whole world became industrialized then certainly someone has to be feeding the farmers who are producing enormous amounts of foods, especially corn which is in almost every food item we consume and ingest today. Then, who's feeding us and the farmers?! Well, it's not a mystery anymore if we go back to the United States and more specifically during Richard Nixon presidency in 1971.

A political deal was done in the early 70s when the United States was devastated during the Vietnam War. The price of food rapidly increased and never seen before at least for the last forty years. People were filling the streets across the nation protesting not only against the war in Vietnam and South East Asia but also, against the high food prices.

Nixon was facing a hard time with the protestors, the food prices and the situation in the country. Additionally, he needed the support of the farmers, and the farmers agreed but with some conditions. In 1971 Nixon assigned this job to Earl Butz, who served as Secretary of Agriculture under Presidents Richard Nixon and Gerald Ford. The decision was made in 1971 and it had a significant effect on agriculture and a great influence on the food, even the kind of which we eat today.

Earl Butz was born in Albion, Indiana, and brought up on a dairy farm in Noble County, Indiana. His background of being raised on a farm gave him some great advantages in dealing with the farmers and he knew exactly how to work and communicate with them despite his academic background. His ability to relate to the farmers served his goal in transforming agriculture from a small farm to a massive production industry providing cheap food on a widespread national scale across the country, and later exporting worldwide.

Earl Butz encouraged the farmers to grow and produce more. His idea was to get the farmers to farm wherever they could without leaving an inch of land unproductive or unfarmed. His motto was "get big or get out". This led many small farmers to go out of business and that was the birth of a bigger, stronger and fatter industrial farming empire, and later to oversizing people, their plates and certainly the waist line.

After the huge production of corn started, the farmers had farmed every inch they had, planting fence row to fence row as Butz suggested. The harvest season started and the amount of the harvested corn was enormous to the point of becoming the feed of the cheap beef flooding the supermarkets. Butz's plan didn't stop there. His vision was greater and to even grow more, that's what he told the farmers to do.

To the farmers, it was a good way to prosper and also to stay in the game especially during a time where the food prices were so high and leaving the farmers no choice but to farm big to survive. Butz told the farmers "adapt or die" believing that they should be thinking of themselves as agribusinesses rather than farmers. Butz's famous motto was "either get big or get out, grow or go". No farmer wanted to be out of the game especially after finding themselves forced to be in the competition or they would be facing the same fate as the smaller farmers faced - "out". Out of the game meant out of business and that's not what the farmers wanted at any rate. Farmers started to grow more, and the more they grew the more they sold just as Butz' planned. He also planned to introduce a new product which would change everything for a very long time, and he succeeded.

In the 1970s, Japanese scientists discovered a process which could convert corn-starch into an alternative sweetener called "High Fructose Corn Syrup" HFCS. According to the Center for Health and Nutrition Research, Department of Nutrition University of California, this type of sweetener contains 55% fructose and 45% glucose, which makes it essentially as sweet as natural honey. By the 1980s, this industrial sweet corn syrup replaced table sugar and it became the number one champion sweetener for its cheap price and availability. That's how Earl Butz changed the American diet and oversized the world.

In an article published in 2004, the US National Library of Medicine National Institutes of Health states that "Obesity is a major epidemic, but its causes are still unclear. In this article, we investigate the relations between the intake of high-fructose corn syrup (HFCS) and the development of obesity. We analyzed food consumption patterns by using US Department of Agriculture food consumption tables from 1967 to 2000. The consumption of HFCS has increased by 1000 percent between 1970 and 1990. It far exceeded the changes in intake of any other food or food group. HFCS now represents more than 40 percent of caloric sweeteners added to foods and beverages and is the sole caloric sweetener in soft drinks in the United States. Our most conservative estimate of the consumption of HFCS indicates a daily average of 132 kcal for all Americans aged > or = 2 y, and the top 20% of consumers of caloric sweeteners ingest 316 kcal from HFCS/d. The increased use of HFCS in the United States mirrors the rapid increase in obesity. The digestion, absorption and metabolism of fructose differ from that of glucose. Hepatic metabolism of fructose favors de novo lipogenesis. In addition, unlike glucose, fructose does not stimulate insulin secretion or enhance Leptin production. Because insulin and Leptin act as key afferent signals in the regulation of food intake and body weight, this suggests that dietary fructose may contribute to increased energy intake and weight gain. Furthermore, calorically sweetened beverages may enhance caloric overconsumption. Thus, the increase in consumption of HFCS has a temporal relation to the epidemic of obesity, and the overconsumption of HFCS in calorically sweetened beverages may play a role in the epidemic of obesity."

Since the 1980s corn syrup - which has no nutritional value but adverse metabolic effects, huge amount of calories and the high risk of getting type two diabetes etc. - started to stretch its path to be in food products, and today it is in almost any product you can find on the shelf of your local or big supermarket stores. Anywhere in the world and in almost every food you eat or drink regardless what it is. Take an example of a hamburger meal. The beef is fed on corn, the bread you eat is made with corn syrup used as preservatives to make it last longer. The sauce on your burger has also corn sweetener syrup, the fries are deep fried in corn oil and last but not the least; the soda drink regardless of its brand or flavor it's made with corn syrup as a sweetener (HFCS)! That was only an example of one meal and the list goes on and on with almost all food and drink products, thanks to Butz.

More about sweeteners and sugar will be in a later chapter "sugar the sweet toxin".

Monsanto:

If we want to start asking the question of who is feeding us or the farmers, it would not be fair not to mention the infamous Monsanto. The huge multinational chemical and agricultural biotechnology corporation. Wherever I turned to in the last several years researching about foods, seeds and genetics, I found the name

Monsanto always showing up everywhere. Monsanto is one of the most controversial corporations in the world, because of its production to genetically engineered seeds, and Monsanto is the world's leading producer of Roundup®, an herbicide with the active ingredient glyphosate. Monsanto is also the largest production corporation of genetically engineered (GE) seeds on the planet, accounting for over 90% of the GE seeds planted globally in 2003.

Monsanto introduced a genetically modified product (Roundup Ready Soybeans) resistant to Roundup. The first crops introduced were soybeans, followed by corn in 1998. "Roundup Ready" crops greatly improved a farmer's ability to control weeds, since glyphosate could be sprayed in the fields without harming their crops. However, Roundup turned up to kill everything except the genetically modified crop. The seeds are engineered to resist the Roundup herbicide. Also, Roundup Ready seeds are genetically modified to withstand the herbicide toxicity. This is also the primary purpose of all genetically modified seeds, to resist pests, drought and most importantly pesticide and herbicide. In simple terms, if the seed is "Roundup Ready" then it will survive Monsanto's glyphosate herbicide while killing everything else around it.

Throughout its history, Monsanto has developed chemical products which have eventually become controversial or have been banned, including DDT, Agent Orange, Bovine Growth Hormone, and PCBs. The animals have been feeding on unnatural foods such as the GM corn and Growth Hormones has made them grow faster to be sold faster. Let us not forget the antibiotics given to the animals to avoid getting sick and dying so the industry can grow more profit - more about that will be detailed in a later chapter. The food chain is running faster and bigger by the day but sadly it's not running better in our favor.

"Don't believe everything you hear: Real eyes, Realize, Real lies."

- Tupac Shakur

"A lie is half-truth is the darkest of all lies."
- Alfred lord Tennyson

Chapter 3
GMO/GE food V.S Organic Food

G.M.O. or G.E. foods now being scientifically engineered are flooding our food supplies in almost every product from the seed and soil to the stomach. G.M.O stands for Genetically Modified Organisms and G.E. stands for Genetically Engineered. These are terms to indicate that food, meat or plant food sources have been genetically engineered by a laboratory process where scientists take a gene from a species and force it into the DNA of another or different species. The implanted genes may come from bacteria, viruses, insects, animals or even humans. Because this involves the transfer of genes, GMOs are also known as "transgenic" organisms. This process may be called either Genetic Engineering (GE) or Genetic Modification (GM). They are one and the same but GMO does NOT mean God Move Over so we can take your place!

It takes very little research to understand how dangerous and harmful G.E. foods are and how that food shouldn't be in our diets. Every single independent study that has been conducted on GMO food indicates that GMO food causes infertility, holes in the gastrointestinal tract (GI tract), damages organs, immune system failure, multiple organ system failure and accelerates ageing. Also, studies have shown that genetically modified (GM) foods can leave materials behind as residuals inside us, which possibly may cause long-term problems and most likely might affect our genes. That means "you are what you eat" is true and it's as scientific as it gets.

A cutting-edge new research conducted by Chinese researchers' shows, microscopic RNA (Ribonucleic Acid) [which stores genetic information and transfer the genetic code needed for the creation of proteins from the nucleus to the ribosome] in the plants or food you eat when it enters your body is capable of affecting the expression of your genes! This also means that if the foods you eat is genetically modified (unnaturally genetically enhanced), it will affect your genes unnaturally and mess up your genetic information and stop certain genes from being expressed. An example of this process is when Monsanto modifies the plants on the genetic level, the plant is no longer the source of food that your genes have adjusted to since thousands of years ago. These new genetic codes of the modified plant will mess up your genes and that will cause lots of complications when it's consumed.

On the other hand, when GMO corns are also fed to cows and animals, the GMO corn will also affect that animals and their meet, milk and eggs, which eventually we consume. This process will change the course of nature but before those changes occur, many diseases, illness, epidemics and pandemics will emerge. Let's not forget the Avian Influenza — known informally as avian flu or birds' flu in 2003, the swine flu or pig's flu the one which took a different genetic form in 1997 and the Bovine spongiform encephalopathy (BSE) commonly known as mad cow disease in the late 1980s and early 1990s. What did really happen to those animals? Think about how many people consumed those animals, consumed their milk and consumed their eggs before we knew those pandemics even existed? What if there is a common link between those three pandemics and the GMO seeds? The fact is, most of those pandemics occurred in the late 1980s which are the same time GM seeds officially started these changes. Most of the meat and fast foods you live on today is meat fed on corn, especially cows and chickens. Although, cows and chickens are not naturally meant to eat corn - but because GM corn is cheap, available and make the animals grow faster and heavier, the Growth Hormones and antibiotics involved in their industrialized farming ends up on your plate. If animals can't take such food what makes you so sure that you could?!

GMO from a different perspective

According to the World Health Organization (WHO), genetically modified organisms (GMOs) are "organisms of which their genetic material (DNA) has been altered in such a way that it does not occur naturally." That means scientists add, change or enhance a gene from one organism into another to "improve" or change the organism. Nevertheless, is it safe? And if it is safe, to what extent and is there any downsides or side effects of this process? The question is easy but the answer seems complicated depending on who you ask. A bio-engineer would tell you yes if it's done right, while a medical doctor would tell you it is totally harmful. And if you research through the lab report results regarding the safety of GMOs on humans, earthlings and the environment, how much would you trust the results if they said: "Yes, GMO foods are safe." Would you trust the test results were not tampered with, unbiased, and not being bought by the corporations? Or deep in your mind, there is a voice screaming about whether the results of those tests are genuine, honest and legitimate? Keep in mind that very powerful corporations own the GMO industries as well as many labs. History is full of evidence of powerful people having tampered with history itself!

I've been asked before what do I think, GMO's or natural organic foods? My answer is and as always will be; I'm a person of science but I'm not a scientist, biotech or bioengineer to give a professional opinion about the safety of GMO, but I can present researches done by experts in this field regarding this matter. Many of them say that GMOs cause cancers, as have displayed some horrible tumors, were developed on rats those of which were fed GMO, herbicide or pesticide foods. These tests were conducted by Monsanto and other experts. On the contrary, I can tell you that there is also a difference between the words natural and nature. Natural is good but nature can be very cruel sometimes, especially if we temper with it! When we start tampering with nature, nature will make sure to get rid of us in one way or another, to regain its natural nature or balance. Therefore, nature and natural are one thing but with two different identities! GMO is not natural, based on its synthetic engineered nature, as well as the definition of the World Health Organization (WHO) defining that genetically modified organisms (GMOs) are "organisms in which the genetic material (DNA) have been altered in such a way that it does not occur naturally." Other organizations have their own definition of GMO but they are all similar. GMO is NOT natural nor can fit in nature based on its biohazards effect on humans, animals and nature, especially when it comes to its biohazard wastes. However, I'll briefly share with you this research from the two points of view and you decide what is good for you and your family.

According to the US National Library of Medicine National Institutes of Health "The Food and Drug Administration's (FDA's) 1992 policy statement granted genetically engineered foods presumptive GRAS (generally recognized as safe) status." That means the FDA granted genetically engineered foods as safe for the public and the environment! Also, the GRAS status granted by the FDA seems to indicate that the genetically engineered foods industry is not obligated to conduct long-term safety studies. Moreover, let's see how GMO works starting with corn.

The majority of the world's corn now produces its own pesticide: BT delta endotoxin. When pests eat the corn, the pesticide dissolves the walls of their stomach. Furthermore, here's how it works, according to Prof. Ric Bessin, Extension Entomologist, University of Kentucky College of Agriculture, "Within minutes, the protein binds to the gut wall and the insect stops feeding. Within hours, the gut wall breaks down and normal gut bacteria invade the body cavity. The insect dies of septicemia as bacteria multiply in the blood." That means the BT toxins is killing the pests but we're also ingesting the same toxin! Till now the industry has always argued that if these toxins were eaten by animals or humans they would be destroyed in the stomach and pass out of the body, thus causing no harm. However, a new study was carried out by independent doctors at the Department of Obstetrics and Gynecology, at the University of Sherbrooke Hospital Centre in Quebec, Canada. The study shows that BT toxin was detected in the bloodstream of 69% of the population tested. For pregnant women, this number was much higher reaching 93%. So, we can't get rid of it after all as claimed and argued!

Another recent study by a Norwegian professor Åshild Krogdahl matched two groups of animals such as rats, mice, pigs and salmons. One had been fed GM corn and the other non-GM corn. The result was noticed 90 days later, the animals that were fed the GM corn had put on more weight (speaking of obesity!) and had changes in their immune system. The same effect occurred if the animals were fed meat that was raised on GM corn. According to Professor Åshild Krogdahl, Norwegian School of Veterinary Science (NVH), states "the ones who had fed on GM corn were slightly larger, they ate slightly more, their intestines had a different microstructure, they were less able to digest proteins, and there were some changes to their immune system. Blood samples also showed some change in the blood." And "If the same effect applies to humans, how would it impact on people eating this type of corn over a number of years, or even eating meat from animals feeding on this corn? I don't wish to sound alarmist, but it is an interesting phenomenon and worth exploring further." That might explain the global obesity, but it's not the only reason, though, it's one of several factors. BT corn started gaining popularity in the late 90's.

This is when childhood obesity in the US skyrocketed to an all-time high.

GMO and children digestive allergy

The obvious child obesity in the 1990s in the U.S was accompanied with another medical issue that is worth mentioning. This was the digestive and food allergies which children had developed between the years 1997 – 2007. The Centers for Disease Control and Prevention (CDC), National Center for Health Statistics, stated:

"•In 2007, approximately 3 million children under 18 years (3.9%) were reported to have a food or digestive allergy in the previous 12 months.

•From 1997 to 2007, the prevalence of reported food allergy increased 18% among children under 18 years.

•Children with food allergy are two to four times more likely to have other related conditions such as asthma and other allergies, compared with children without food allergies.

•From 2004 to 2006, there were approximately 9,500 hospital discharges per year with a diagnosis related to food allergy among children under 18 years."

Looking at the conclusion of the Centers For Disease Control and Prevention (CDC) above especially from the year 1997 to 2007, food allergy with children increased 18% and relating what Professor Åshild Krogdahl stated in regards to the study of the two animal groups that were fed GMO and the other that were not fed GMO. Now notice the links in Professor Åshild Krogdahl statement about the animal group that was fed GMO. Professor Åshild Krogdahl's statement:

"The ones that were fed on GM corn were slightly larger, they ate slightly more, their intestines had a different microstructure, they were less able to digest proteins, and there were some changes to their immune system. Blood samples also showed some change in the blood."

Furthermore, the allergic reaction process, according to U.S. Department of Health and Human Services, National Institutes of Health (NIAID, NIH) is as follows:

"The first time you are exposed to a food allergen, your immune system makes specific immunoglobulin E (IgE) antibodies to that allergen. IgE antibodies circulate through your blood and attach to types of immune cells called mast cells and basophils. Mast cells are found in all body tissues, especially in your nose, throat, lungs, skin, and GI (gastrointestinal) tract. Basophils are found in your blood and also in tissues that have become inflamed because of an allergic reaction."

Let me put this in simpler terms so we can all make sense of it - food allergies as stated above occur when the immune system misidentifies food/s as an intruder/s, the most common intruders to the immune system are bacteria. Now, if we start putting bacteria gene into plants (on the plant's genetic level as the plant's DNA), birds and animals eat those plants such as corn, and we eat the plant (corn, cereal, HFCS sweeteners etc.) and the animals (cows, chickens etc.). It is possible that the immune system may start to get confused about what's food and what's bacterium from what we're eating - plants and animals! If you remember above what Professor Åshild Krogdahl stated about the animal group which were fed GMO:

"If the same effect applies to humans, how would it impact people eating this type of corn over a number of years, or even eating meat from animals feeding on this corn? I don't wish to sound alarmist, but it is an interesting phenomenon and worth exploring further." And I also don't wish to sound and alarmist and I also believe this phenomenon is worth to be further explored especially because GMO and GE mean Genetically Modified Food and Genetically Engineered means the food we eat is altered and engineered on the genetic and on the very DNA level. How would our genes or DNA deal and react with this? And is it worth the risk?!

Allergies and reactions related to GMOs

On the subject of allergies and the reaction process, according to (NIAID, NIH), consequently, I recalled a report of an event which occurred in spring of 1999. According to a Report to the Administrator, Pesticide Control Act, Ministry of Environment, Lands and Parks, Province of British Columbia, a bacterial pest control product called Foray 48B (manufactured by Abbott Laboratories), was applied by aircraft (aerial spray) to spray BT over regions of Vancouver and Washington State to control the gypsy moth population. The spray event led to 500 people reporting adverse reactions. The majority complained of allergy or flu-like symptoms and six others were hospitalized for severe allergic reactions or asthma flare-ups. Farmers and workers exposed to BT sprays have reported eye, nose, throat, skin and respiratory irritations (just as the allergic reaction process according to the NIAID, NIH mentioned above "tissues, especially in your nose, throat, lungs, skin"). Authorities have cautioned against the effects of the spray for years warning - "People with compromised immune systems or preexisting allergies may be particularly susceptible to the effects of BT." (Same reaction symptoms as mentioned in the allergic reaction process according to the (NIAID, NIH).

According to the American Academy of Environmental Medicine (AAEM), "several animal studies indicate serious health risks associated with genetically modified foods". These health risks include Immune

Impairment, Infertility, lung damage, vitamin deficient, premature ageing, damaged insulin regulation, liver, kidney, heart and spleen dysfunction, higher rate of mortality and cancer.

Are GMOs dangerous? And do GMOs cause cancer?

Cancers related to GMOs are a very serious and controversial subject due to the shadows clouding tests results from many sides by very big and powerful corporations, politicians, media and scientists. For example, according to a report analysis by the Food & Water Watch indicates that in just over a decade, the food and agriculture biotechnology industry has spent more than $572 million in campaign contributions and lobbying expenses. One aim of this extreme lobbying effort is to prevent GM food labelling and keep Americans ignorant about the contents of their food, while GMO labelling has existed in Europe since 1997.

It is also claimed that so far there are no reported human clinical trials confirming the devastating effects of the Bt-toxin on human health, which may or may not be possible. As with any research, you expect to get debunkers doubting independent studies, reports and research. Then I personally ask; what makes a researcher connected to the same people who are running the show more credible than an independent researcher who runs independently, especially when there are over half a billion dollars spent in campaigning and lobbying? Nevertheless, regarding the claim "there is no reported clinical trials confirming the devastating effects of the Bt-toxin on human health". Well, there is a specific type of Bt-toxin called Cry1Ab that is already widespread in humans. I have referred to this earlier in this chapter regarding the Canadian researchers who found high levels of the toxin in pregnant and non-pregnant women whose diet consisted of foods such as genetically modified corn, soy and potatoes. Bt-toxin was present in 93% of maternal blood samples, 80% of fetal blood samples and 67% of non-pregnant women's blood samples.

However, just to be fair here, if GMOs trigger or cause cancers, then GMOs wouldn't be the only factors causing cancers. Also, based on an extensive research about cancers and the causes of cancers, I've found that there are many factors that will lead to cancers. Those factors will be discussed here in greater details in a later chapter.

Consequently, while I was researching and collecting some materials, I came across some really horrifying photos, painful even to look at – the photos can be easily found online. The photos showed rats had developed huge tumors on them, claiming to be a new study that shows Monsanto's genetically modified corn and Roundup© herbicide causes negative health effects in those rats. The study is alarming and is raising questions about the safety of GMOs. It was released in September 2012 involving the publication of an experiment conducted by a group led by a French scientist Dr. Gilles-Eric Séralini, who has been a professor of molecular biology. The journal became very controversial and then again the shadow clouded the results when the journal was withdrawn by the publisher which supposedly showed that genetically modified maize causes tumors in rats.

Later, a wave of biotech-industry criticism had risen and "experts" said the study led by Dr. Séralini was grossly unscientific, its methods were unprofessional and Dr. Seralini was biased against GMOs from the beginning. Obviously, Monsanto didn't like Seralini and surely the journal was withdrawn, could be due to the very powerful people behind the GMO industry and their influence on the media and politics.

On a side note, more than two decades ago, the U.S. Food and Drug Administration (FDA) granted GMOs "generally regarded as safe" (GRAS) status. That means the GMO industry had no obligation to conduct long-term safety studies. It's claimed by scientists that GMOs does not have "acute" effects, but the important question is what about "chronic" affects, those that come on progressively and can't easily be tied to just one cause? The French study is believed to be the most comprehensive GMO safety assessment ever conducted that addresses this concern.

The study involved 200 rats with two years lifespan as it was the life expectancy of the species of rat involved in this particular research. The longest study had lasted 240 days in previous studies. The researchers were investigating the effect of eating Monsanto's Roundup©-Ready corn (and any Roundup© herbicide traces that may come with it) on rats' health. The rats were divided into 10 groups: Three had part of their standard diet replaced at varying levels with Roundup©-Ready corn that had been treated with Roundup© in the field; three received the same feed protocol, but with untreated Roundup©-Ready corn; three ate no GM corn but had tiny amounts of Roundup© herbicide in their drinking water, and one controlled group ate two-thirds standard rat chow (such as foods and grubs) and one-third non-GM corn. Each group contained 10 females and 10 males.

According to the researchers, the results showed "severe adverse health effects, including mammary tumors and kidney and liver damage, leading to premature death". This indicated that it was from Roundup©-Ready corn and Roundup© herbicide. The health issues on the rats and the sickness affecting nearly all of them showed after 90 days. Researches also said that by the end of the study 50 – 80% of the female rats had developed large tumors, compared with 30 percent developing tumors in the controlled group. The result in males wasn't less horrifying. The male rats showed liver congestion and necrosis were 2.5 to 5.5 times higher than in the group which didn't receive GM corn and/or Roundup©, and there were 1.3 to 2.3 times more occurrences of kidney disease.

The result overall concluded - among the rats which received GM corn and/or Roundup©, up to 50 percent of males and 70 percent of females died prematurely, compared with only 30 percent and 20 percent in the group which didn't receive GM corn and/or Roundup©.

However, the GMO industry and scientists who support GMOs were questioning the study and doubted its credibility. Regardless, if the GMO industry and its supporting scientists doubt the study and its findings, critics of GMOs and others including Dr. Michael Hansen, a Ph.D. and a senior scientist at Consumers Union and an expert on GMO research still has concerns about GMOs. Dr. Hansen explains in an interview with Steve Curwood in December 6, 2013, at loe.org "while the new study was longer and better designed than any of the industry GMO safety studies, the sample size of 10 males and 10 females per group was too small to draw conclusions from." He Dr. Hansen also said, "However, that while the individual comparisons may not be statistically significant because of sample size, the results still paint a troubling picture. The study made 54 comparisons between treated rats and controlled rats and in all but four, the treated rats showed worse outcomes. That's suggestive that there's something going on and that there should be further research." Dr. Hansen also added, "A possible reason the researchers didn't use a greater number of rats to get more robust results is because multiyear rat studies are extremely expensive."

The story has been caved in as usual into the unknown since late 2012 and has never seen a clear sky since! But one question still remain, If the publishing journal didn't have something important or it proves that GMO didn't have anything to hide, then why was it withdrawn?

"Any politician or scientist who tells you these products are safe is either very stupid or lying."

- David Suzuki

"I always wonder, how we can eat something was farmed by people wearing hazmat suits and call it food?!"

- Adam Musselli

Chapter 4
Why Are We Getting Fatter?

There are many factors leading to weight problems and other related health issues, reaching the highest level of obesity ever recorded in history. But why is this happening to us? Is it all from eating and being lazier? Or are there any other reasons causing this pandemic of obesity?!

Obesity has been around since there were people, before the fast and junk food, before all the GMO/processed food and even before forcing the cattle and chickens to grow faster and bigger.

Obesity is a part of human's physiology because people who store energy are more likely to be able to survive for a longer time during periods of adversities, migrations, starvation and famine. It is a natural condition for the human's body. However, it is unnatural for humans on a global scale to become unbelievably overweight or obese in only a few decades. That's a reason for this phenomenon to be considered as a pandemic rather than epidemic. Pandemic is on a global level and epidemic is only on a regional or national level, and since obesity is now global this makes it a pandemic phenomenon. It is absurd and farfetched to believe that we got to this level of obesity simply because we became lazier. Think of it this way, if this is the case then how can we explain the obesity among infants who are only 5 or 6 months old? I believe, as many other professionals in this field that this pandemic of obesity isn't only about eating healthy foods and exercising. And if so, how about young children and 6 months old infants, they don't diet or exercise. Does that mean the obese 6-month-old infant is lazy? This is clearly not all based on personal responsibilities!

If you ask any dietician or nutritional expert about what is the first thing a dietician learns at college or university. They will tell you "a calorie is a calorie no matter if you get that calorie from a strawberry or if you get it from French fries, it is still a calorie. If you eat more than what you can't burn you'll gain weight, and if you eat less than what you burn you'll lose weight", that is what most dieticians tell you. However, this is not true and it doesn't work because a calorie is not a calorie, and the only answer for that equation is, sadly, there is none. There is no specific reason to tell you why people started gaining so much weight in the last three decades because there are too many reasons. Such as the easy access to food, the high fructose corn syrup, the anti-biotic medications we're taking (especially from animal products), the oestrogens (especially from plastic), different hormones and hormone's mimickers, and many other factors play a role in this global obesity. It is definitely not only one reason, but the major reason is our food environment as you'll later learn in later chapters.

Our lifestyle and how things have become easier for our convenience also plays a major role in weight gain, such as driving instead of walking or even simpler things such as washing a plate in the dish washer instead of by hand, doing online shopping and ordering foods by a click of a button. Many things have been invented for us and for our benefits to save us time and energy. But the question is, are those things that are supposed to be made for our convenience really serving us right?

There are lots of changes happened in the last few decades, especially our interaction with foods on many different levels. For example; tens of thousands of food items enter the markets every year. And our sleep patterns have been interrupted due to many reasons such as TV, the Internet, work, stress etc. Also what has been fed to the animals and other food sources which people consume, such as anti-biotic, the soil for crops and plants, pesticides, GMOs and others.

There was a debate in the late 1970s between fat and sugar which was prepared by the staff of the select committee on nutrition and human needs. United States Senate in 95th Congress, 1st session in February 1977 titled "Dietary Goals for the United States" stated on page 12 section 2 to "reduce overall fat consumption from approximately 40 – 30 energy intake". However, everyone did it but the total consumptions of calories and specifically carbohydrates and more specifically sugar has reached a very high level, which led the masses to the metabolic syndrome imbalances. Even till this day, it's almost impossible to buy any packaged food from any supermarket without getting a big amount of extra sugar in the food. The extra sugar is going to be toxic to our metabolism, and the more we consume it the more we want it because it's addictive. Also, there is no doubt about the low fat, diet food, and drink beverages which contain lots of artificial and added sugars, especially Aspartame.

Moreover, here's a brief explanation about Aspartame. According to the FDA, Aspartame is just an artificial sweetener, despite the fact that it was banned by the FDA twice, but now it is legal and considered as safe by the FDA. Nevertheless, many top researchers in this field have done many studies showing that Aspartame is a sweet poison, and some studies have shown - there are over 92 different health side effects associated with aspartame consumption. Aspartame is an addictive, excitoneurotoxic, carcinogenic, genetically engineered drug and adjuvant that damages the mitochondria or the powerhouse of the cells and interacts with drugs and vaccines. Despite the dangers of that sweetener in light - low-fat food and drink products, you'll find the same amount of calories in both products, and sometimes more calories in the low-fat or light products! More about Aspartame will be in later chapters "Sugar the Sweet Toxin and Suggestions".

Nowadays almost every item you purchase contains some sweeteners such as Corn Sweeteners - very high in artificial sugar. The problem isn't fat which is driving the world toward obesity, the problem is sugar, sweeteners and carbohydrates! You go to the market to purchase a diet food product, and you'll find the diet product has 2 grams of fat reduced and 10 – 20 grams of extra carbohydrates added on which is mostly sugar. The amount of calories will also increase because of the increased amount of sugar/carbohydrate and that is the problem. It is not fat but it's the sugar! That is why people keep wondering why they are not losing weight although they are on major well-known diet and low-fat programs.

The next step from sugar, carbs, and obesity is the diseases caused by them. If you're wondering what are the main diseases of obesity, then wonder no more. They are type two diabetes, Lipid problems (blood fat), hypertension and heart disease. Those are called The Metabolic Syndrome, which is the disorder of energy utilization and storage. However, those four aren't the only diseases of obesity. We have several others that are also believed to be closely associated with obesity such as fatty liver disease (non-alcoholic which now affects one-third of all Americans), Polycystic Ovarian Syndrome (now affects 10% of all women), cancer and dementia, based on the Journal of Clinical Endocrinology & Metabolism.

It's believed that these diseases are caused or at least triggered by obesity and most likely to be true. It is also believed that obesity uses these diseases and sets itself as a precursor for these diseases. According to an article, the National Institutes of Health, it indicates that 20% of obese people have a totally normal cellular metabolism and they will live a normal age. 40% of normal non-obese people have those same chronic metabolic diseases and will die of them. These people will die from metabolic malfunction not from obesity. The total of that equation is 60% in the United State only! If you add all those diseases, the medical cost will be 75% of the global health care cost, as you will see in the detailed figures later.

Furthermore, on the 19th of September 2011, the United Nations Secretary-General announced:: "non-communicable disease that chronic, metabolic disease (type 2 diabetes, heart disease, hypertension, cancer and dementia) now pose a bigger threat to the developing world than what did acute infectious disease that includes HIV". That's outrageous, when you think of the developing countries have a bigger problem now with obesity and diabetes than they do with cholera, malaria, HIV and other infectious diseases. Here's another question, is this a mere coincidences or there is a conspiracy have been pulled out behind the dark curtains? We'll also get to that in a specific chapter.

The mind and the stomach

In addition to the Chronic Metabolic Diseases and the reduction in calories. Surely, doctors and nutritionists love to tell their clients the golden motto of every nutritionist "eat less and exercise more". Despite how ridiculous this may sound but in reality is this motto does not work. At least not with the first part of it "eat less".

The reason why "eat less and exercise more" doesn't work is because there is one new hormone that has been discovered called "Leptin". According to the National Institutes of Health – US National Library of Medicine, explains Leptin is a hormone that goes from your fat cells to your brain and tells your brain that your stomach now is full now or had enough food and you can start burning energy at an average rate. This is a great hormone which God /nature provided us with to maintain our health and prevent us from the illnesses and diseases related to food and obesity. This very useful hormone Leptin limits what you eat and also it lets you exercise and burn the energy and calories you had from your meals. This hormone also makes you feel good about exercising, because it gives you the feeling of you want to exercise, or that exercising is fun. Obviously because of the calories burning mechanism which Leptin is designed/evolved to produce.

However, overweight and obese people have a higher level of Leptin because they have a higher level of fats stored in their bodies and Leptin comes from the fat cells. But, if Leptin was doing its assigned and regular job then there wouldn't be any overweight and/or obesity problem! So, what is the valid explanation for having a high level of Leptin, still eating too much, and maybe not exercising, while fat is not being burnt as it should be?! The answer is simple, leptin is not doing its job. And that is called Leptin Resistance, which is the answer for overweight problems and obesity. This is the obesity Holy Grail which we're all searching for "Leptin Resistance". I wonder how Leptin used to work normally if not perfectly three decades ago, and now it does not? Researchers have found a very significant answer to the reason that causes Leptin Resistance, and the answer is simply "Insulin". Insulin is one of the main causes of obesity - that is if not the major one.

What is Insulin?

Many people have heard of the word "Insulin" and many people know that insulin is the diabetes hormone. I'll simply explain how it works in the body and its direct relation to obesity. A diabetic person takes shots of insulin when needed to lower their blood sugar. Let's say their blood sugar is high as 300 mg/dL (16.6 mmol/L), now the diabetic is given an Insulin shot. Their blood sugar goes down from 300 mg/dL to 100 mg/dL (5.5 mmol/L). Now you might be thinking that is great so far reducing the blood sugar from 300 mg/dL down to 100 mg/dL which is

200 mg/dL (11 mmol/L) less. But the question is; where are those 200 points now and where did they go to? Those 200 mg/dL were in the blood and now they are not. They must have gone somewhere! Well, they went to fat for storage, simply because insulin returns to its origin (fat cells). Therefore, insulin makes fat and more insulin means more fat. That's how insulin drives to weight gain and weight gain drives to obesity.

A simple way to further explain how it works technically and similarly as Prof. Robert H. Lustig, University of California, San Francisco, explains it; I'm going to take you as an example. You are an average healthy person. You eat 2000 calories a day and you burn 2000 calories a day, and you feel good as it's all balanced and nice for a normal day. In this way, you're not going to gain weight or lose weight. You are just going to stay the same because simply you burn what you eat and you have nothing left from the 2000 calories you ate to be stored. However, now let's try something else as a little experiment. Let's say I put an IV drip in your arm and I'm going to be with you all the time, and every time you reach for food to eat I'm going to pump you with some extra Insulin in that IV which you didn't want or simply your body didn't need. I'm going to keep pumping you with Insulin, same as what they do to diabetic people. Now, it's a new day and you start eating 2000 calories just as before, but now because of the extra Insulin I'm pumping you with 500 calories of 2000 will go straight to fat before you even had the chance to burn it. You are now 500 calories heavier and if you stand on the scale you'll weigh a 7th of a pound more which around 55 grams heavier every day whether you like it or not because of the Insulin I have pumped you with. This calculation is based on the 9 calories are the equivalent to 1 gram of fat equation, which will result in 55 grams of fat in the 500 calories. Furthermore, it's true that you ate 2000 calories, you also lost 500 calories to your fat and now you have 1500 calories to burn, however, your body wants to burn 2000 calories because that's what feels right and good to your body. The things that would drive you to burn more energy make you feel good such as exercise, caffeine etc. On the other hand, things that wouldn't drive you to burn energy make you feel lousy such as starvation and hypothyroidism (when the thyroid gland doesn't make enough thyroid hormone - which is the hormone that runs the body's metabolism). That means the number of calories you burn and how good you feel are the same. Now you only have 1500 calories to burn but your body wants to burn 2000 calories and that is what we call "starvation". This is why you feel tired, moody, and lousy or you don't feel like doing any exercise and of course you feel hungry. As you know, we all live in a world where we have very easy access to food. What do you think you would do when you feel like that? Of course, eat back the 500 calories! So, now instead of eating 2000 calories, you'll be eating 2500 calories. That means you increased your food intake to make up or compensate for the effects of the extra insulin. The game keeps getting worse because I'm still pumping you with extra insulin and now 100 calories of those 500 calories you have newly added will go straight to fat and now you're 600 calories heavier which is 63 grams a day heavier on the scale, and you have 1900 calories to burn and you still don't feel good. So, you go to the doctor or nutritionist and say "doc, every time I step on the scale I weigh more and I don't feel good. What is going on and why am I fat"? And the doctor will look at you and tell you their golden quote "well, you're fat because you're lazy. You eat too much and don't exercise enough that's why you're fat"! Well, the doctor is right, you're eating too much and not burning or exercising enough and maybe you're lazy but NOT because you want to or chose to! It's because you have to. A biochemical drive is set up by the amount of extra insulin that I have pumped you with and that explains what has been happening in the last few decades. Moreover, it's true you're not being pumped with insulin, but the changes of the global food industry got you to make it yourself. Insulin is being pumped in almost every food product you consume. If you're wondering about why your leptin is not working? Recently, researchers found that insulin blocks leptin in the brain and that drives you to feel hungry. So, the higher your Insulin goes the more energy you store and the more hungry you get. That's the sick cycle of food consumption and we're all voluntarily and/or involuntarily became a part of it. Weight gain, disease and illness are all being brought to you by the excess Insulin from non-other than the global food industry.

Why are we eating more?

I totally believe that everything nature helped to evolve has evolved in a rhythmic way, balanced with its surroundings and environment. Up until us humans temper with it or its nature. This behavior will cause the inequities and surely will backfire on us as well as on other species.

We are naturally equipped with leptin. This leptin acts like a system which allowed us to control our food intake for thousands of years since human evolution. Suddenly, in the last three or four decades, things have gone extremely wrong. How did we do that or how did that happen? The answer can be found in understanding the bio-chemistry of the brain because obviously leptin, which is the starvation signal, is not functioning as it should be along with other factors.

This is how it works - leptin tells your brain that you've had enough food or you're full and you can now burn energy, but when you don't get the leptin signal you're brain thinks you're still hungry.

There is another factor in the reward system and this is how it also works. There is a reward center in your brain is called the Nucleus Accumbens, it's the place where dopamine works. According to the National Centre for Biotechnology Information, dopamine is a neurotransmitter which gives you the feeling of pleasure and goodness. The process of going for more pleasure will cause us to change our dopamine system or pattern and that's one of the main keys of addictions - which is the idea of after stimulating that system frequently over and over again the respecters for the dopamine signals will now down regulate and there will be only a few of them that are left to function as they should be.

The brain of an obese person responds in a different way to food than that of a thin or a person of an average weight. When an obese person sees tangible food, some parts of their brain start to light up rapidly which is the wanting part function in that reward center, but the liking part once the person tastes the food will lose interest because there is no more pleasure or reward being received from it. This is simply as living with an urge you can't satisfy, so people think this inability to achieve or experience the same level of reward and pleasure from the same food that other people are getting is causing people to eat more in order to get that dopamine and the feeling or experience of the reward which they're looking for.

Moreover, now the brain has the fear of missing out on the reward. This causes people to start eating more to get that effect of dopamine which is pleasurable. This process is called tolerance, and now when you pull away from the chemicals that cause the pleasure there will have no dopamine left, and also only a few receptors left which that will lead to withdrawal. Tolerance and withdrawal are the main causes of addiction because we know that happens with nicotine - tobacco addiction as well as alcohol, cocaine, morphine, LSD, heroin and every addictive drug you can think of and it also happens with sugar. According to the US National Library of Medicine National Institutes of Health, there is a research shows specifically that sugar down-regulates the same receptors in the reward center (Nucleus

Accumbens) the same as any addictive drugs, alcohol and tobacco. We also know that more exposure to food might change the way our brain functions and food exposure might also lead to addictions based on the repetitive message getting into the brain when seeing food, food signs, food advertisements and that is getting worse every single day. Now we also know that developing compulsive eating (food addiction) will cause changes in the wiring of the brain, which is the way we think. That's a big concern to know that food is changing the way we're thinking and you'll find out more about that in the "Media and the psychological factor" chapter.

The Genetic Effect

What we are witnessing now is obesity in infants and children. A six or seven-month-old child is already obese! Is this normal and how did it happen? The simplest answer is - fat is passed on to the child before the child was even born, and the way it can be determined is the baby's insulin level before the baby is born. And what determines the baby's insulin is the mother's diet before pregnancy and even before conception, that's how women are shaping the future generations.

There is a very obvious increase in birth weight in the last 25 years on the global scale and also there is an increase in women gaining more weight during pregnancy. The statistic shows that women gained 40 lbs. (18.1 kg) since 1990 to 2005 is 20% according to the Centers for Disease Control and Prevention CDC. This increase will indicate the baby's fat cells and the level of storing fat, those fat cells for the babies are there to be used to store fat and those babies once they are born they are hungry and crying for food whether it's breast feeding, bottle or baby formula. The baby is now programmed to eat and fill those fat cells. Although, even if the child is born small or underweight from an obese mother, that doesn't mean later the child's metabolism won't set to be efficient with calories and cause the child to become obese.

According to a study conducted by the American Academy of Child and Adolescent Psychiatry Studies, a child who is obese between the ages of 10 and 13 has an 80 percent chance of becoming obese as an adult. Also, another study was done by the same academy shows - if one parent is obese, there is a 50 percent chance their children will also be obese. However, when both parents are obese, their children have 80 percent chance of also becoming obese.

There is another concern with young girls and obesity - overweight and obesity are influencing younger ages toward puberty. For example, during the process of puberty for young girls, there is a need for development and maturity, as well as going through their own reproduction, which will perversely influence the calories and the fat in the young girls' system. When girls are obese and also putting on more weight during pregnancy, they already are programming the new generation who are coming out to the world to be obese and with early diseases related to obesity. To prevent this situation from re-occurring and from being transmitted from generation to generation, some intervention must take place starting from fixing the diet not only for mothers who are pregnant or before pregnancy or even fixing the diet for children, but fixing the diet for everyone because the obesity problem is becoming worse as every day passes.

Understanding Carbohydrates

We know so far that obesity leads to many health issues and cancers. Obesity and most of today common health problems were rare 100 years ago when people's diets involved whole grains and high fiber foods. Bad carbohydrates lead to obesity and cancers along with other health issues.

Certainly, our bodies need carbohydrates. Carbohydrates are essential nutrients which are responsible for the production of energy in the body to function, work and exercise, but that depends on the type of carbohydrate we consume. The brain's favorite fuel comes from the glucose provided by the breakdown of the good carbohydrates in our bodies.

There are two types of carbohydrates, the good carbohydrates such as complex and unrefined carbohydrate - which are found in brown rice, whole wheat flour, whole oats, and whole grain pasta. Those carbs are good and we need them as fuel for our bodies to survive.

On the other hand, bad carbohydrates are simple carbohydrates and refined carbohydrates. These can be found in foods such as white sugar, some other sugars, sweeteners in soda and candy, white flour, white rice, corn flour, pasta etc. Refined and simple carbs - are bad and they are designed by manufacturers for longer shelf-life.

The differences between refined and unrefined carbohydrates are simple - according to the National Heart Foundation of Australia position statement; carbohydrates, dietary fiber, glycemic index/load and cardiovascular disease, explain best the differences between the two carbohydrates as follow:

"Non-refined carbohydrate foods are rich in vitamins, minerals and mostly dietary fiber, and include foods like wholegrain breads and cereals (e.g. rice and pasta), legumes, fruit, vegetables and dairy foods."

"Refined carbohydrate foods are highly processed with little or no wholegrain fiber, frequently contain a lot of easily consumed energy (kilojoules) and include foods like confectionery, biscuits, cakes, pastries and high sugar drinks. High sugar drinks may include soft drinks, fruit juices or fruit juice drinks and alcoholic beverages."

Unrefined carbohydrates foods are more recommended due to their high nutritional value. Unrefined carbohydrates take longer to digest because glucose is more slowly absorbed into the body and provides energy over a longer period of time. Unrefined carbohydrates contain plenty of vitamins and minerals which are essential to our health and also contain a very healthy amount of fiber. Fiber helps the body to process waste more efficiently and helps us to feel fuller for a longer period of time. According to the diet recommended by Nutrition and Your Health, Dietary Guidelines for Americans (fifth edition, 2000), "more than 60 percent of our foods should be in the form of complex carbohydrates. Lots of salads, fresh or lightly cooked vegetables, and raw fruits should be primary in this approach. Whole-grain cereals and breads, brown rice and other whole grains, beans, nuts, and seeds - these foods will adequately supply necessary fiber as well as fuel reserves." That means (in moderation) complex carbohydrates the "good carbohydrates" are the foundation of a healthy diet and they are an essential food and energy sources for the brain and body.

Now don't get confused between the word complex and unrefined carbohydrates. Complex carbohydrates can be unrefined which is the "good carbs" as stated above with high fiber and healthy nutritious elements that we need as fuel for our bodies to run. Complex carbohydrates can also be industrially refined as well as the simple carbohydrates which are the "bad carbohydrates" for us.

Refined carbohydrates (the bad carbs) are carbohydrates that have been altered by manufacturers to increase their shelf-life. The refinement process transforms an unrefined carbohydrate (the good carbs) into a refined carbohydrate (the bad carbs) by removing the original natural elements such as fiber, healthy oils, vitamins, and minerals, or more commonly known as "bleaching".

Unfortunately, removing the fiber from these products makes them less nutritious. According to Minnesota Department of Health MDH, indicates, unrefined grains (the good carbs) contain 3 major parts: the germ, the endosperm and the bran. The bran is the key as it is high in fiber and contains the majority of the minerals in the grain. In fact, unrefined complex carbohydrates such as brown rice, whole-wheat flour, whole oats, and whole grain pasta offer the body significantly more fiber, B vitamins (niacin, thiamin and riboflavin), vitamin E, magnesium, potassium, zinc, iron, selenium and iron.

Simple Carbohydrates (bad carbs) are in the simple carbohydrate category. They are made of simple molecules which are easy for your body to breakdown and they deliver sugar to the bloodstream quickly. White sugar and white flour based foods are examples of simple carbohydrates. They breakdown quickly causing a fast spike in blood sugar and that's where you get a rush of energy, and then a big drop and your mood goes right along with it. Also, when too much sugar floods the system all at once, your body can't use it all for energy and converts it to fat. Your body ultimately converts excess sugar into glycogen and then into fat for storage. And worse, constantly overwhelming the cells with high levels of sugar is associated with blood sugar related diseases like hypoglycemia, diabetes, and insulin resistance. However, not all simple carbohydrates are "bad carbs", especially when found in some fruits. Those are nutritious carbs. Fresh fruit gives us enzymes, vitamins, minerals and fiber. The point is to recognize these simple carbohydrates are not so "bad", but are still fast sugars that do not sustain our energy levels in the same way the complex carbohydrates do.

In more simpler terms, the simple white carbs that come from foods such as white sugar, white flour etc. are industrially bleached and are addictive, and made as fast foods to also get you hungry faster to eat more. The simple carbs that come from fruit are good because of the vitamins you get from the fruit itself, but those are not meant to be consumed as a meal. The carbohydrates that you need in a healthy meal are found in whole meal, whole wheat, whole grain, brown rice etc. because they contain a high amount of fiber. Also, beware of some bread and food companies, they dye the bread with a brown color to deceive the consumer as this product is whole meal etc. You need to look at the back of the product and see how much dietary fiber the product contains per serving. More about that will be in the "Suggestions" chapter.

That was an explanation of why we are getting fatter. The story doesn't end here, we barely started. In the following chapters, you'll find other factors are also involved and that will give you a better understanding of the problem we're facing.

"we become what we repeatedly do."

— Sean Covey

"The chains of habit are too light to be felt until they are too heavy to be broken."

— Warren Buffett

Chapter 5

Fast/Junk food

We sadly live in a fast world where everything seems to be progressing faster by the day. Almost every person is busy nowadays in these competitive times where we work many hours and sometimes even multiple jobs. We got to the point of not being able to make the right decision of what and when to eat. Consequently, our gustatory needs got devolved in a sense to acquire a nanny to prepare the food for us and feed us. Sadly, that nanny isn't so wise and seems to care less about our health and wellbeing. How can this nanny be all-wise and care when it's blinded by greed?! This greedy nanny is non-other than the global industrial fast food companies.

Fast food doesn't only mean it is fast to order, cook or eat! Fast food also means it's fast to reach the consumer. The whole production process, sales, delivery, cooking and eating the fast food is fast. However, it doesn't seem fast enough to provide the nutrients we need. Also, it doesn't seem so fast when it comes to burning off this kind of food and metabolize it. Fast food = Fat food = Fast to cause diseases!

The Western diet (which is mostly fast food) has become a very profitable industry in the Western World. It's also being widely exported to the whole world because it's cheap, portable and most importantly it is purposely "designed" to taste really good so people will crave for it. It's easily accessible, almost every street corner has fast food outlets and many of them are now open 24 hours with a drive through. You don't need to do anything to get it, just open your wallet and open your mouth. It seems so easy, on the contrary, the calories you're putting into your system are the hard ones to burn.

We all know that fast and junk foods aren't a healthy choice for us, but do we know why it's hard to avoid them? It is because food companies have mastered the perfect taste sensation, largely a blend of salt, sugar and fat, to keep you coming back for more. They spend millions of dollars on their advertisements and campaigns to keep themselves in your mind. In return - to provide the world with the cheapest and unhealthiest addictive foods. That means with your money, they provide you meals of junk food, food with minimal essential nutrients with a lot of fat, sugar and salt, empty calories such as potato chips fries, a burger and soda drink (those are all addictive). A fast food meal is not a meal; it lacks all the nutrients to be considered as a meal. A meal is meant to satisfy your hunger when you eat it and feel full afterwards. Unlike fast and junk addictive foods, you eat it now and you feel hungry within an hour to go back for more. Also, thinking of enjoying a handful of French fries every now and then isn't going to harm you, but the truth is, anything that goes in your body, especially junk food can have negative and serious physical and emotional consequences.

The empire of fast and junk foods wasn't only designed for adults, but it also targets children and teens. According to a study by the Children's Hospital in Boston, teens aged 13 - 17 were given three types of fast-food meals (all including chicken nuggets, French fries, and soda). In one meal, the teens were served a lot of food at once. In another, a lot of food was served at the same time, but in smaller portions and in the third test meal, a lot of food was served but in smaller portions over a 15-minute break. The researchers found that it didn't seem to matter how much food was served, the teens still took in about half of their daily calorie needed in that one meal. The researchers suggested that certain factors inherent in fast food might promote overeating. Some of them are because it's low in fiber, it's high in palatability (that is why it tastes good), it offers a high number of calories in a small portion, it's high in fat, and it's high in sugar in liquid form. Surely, the individual must take part of the responsibility in bringing about self-discipline and education when it comes to food and eating habits. However, in reality, it's not easy to keep up when those junk food brands and restaurants have a convincing selling proposition where they upgrade your ordered food to include more options or bigger portions for minimum additional fees. This is a strategy to increase sales along with increasing consumer loyalty. But essentially it is the consumer who is paying the bigger price, which is the price of health.

Scientists and doctors say that regular consumption of fast food and reduced physical activity will result in obesity. This seems to be a big issue now since the fast food diet hasn't only become the main food diet in the developed countries, but lately is becoming also the main food diet in many developing countries. The trend of moving away from traditional and home cooked healthy diets in eastern countries are also affected by the fast food and obesity problem.

Some scientists claim that fast food causes obesity by encouraging the sense of intentional overeating. A close explanation to the claim made by scientists explains that fast foods are foods with 150% more high-density energy than any other traditional meal. High-density foods have the tendency to compel people to intake more calories than needed by the body. Fast foods are also known for containing high amounts of sugar, oil, flour and sodium or salt which are all major contributors to obesity and food addiction.

According to Jessica Anderson, RD, diabetes educator "The body can only handle so much at one time," referring to fried and deep-fried fast foods. These are usually the major contributing factors to indigestion and acidity, and also arising of metabolic malfunction from the frequent intake of fast foods, which can result in uncontrolled overeating tendencies that can be a leading cause of weight gain and obesity.

Fried fast foods are mostly fried in saturated or trans-fats. Trans-fats are man-made fats. That can be found on the labels of many manufactured foods. Trans-fat is "partially hydrogenated", it means essentially the manufacturer has added hydrogen to a polyunsaturated fat, making it trans-fat. When fat becomes more saturated, it becomes stiffer as in butter or margarine. Trans-fats are also less likely to go off or expire, and that will give it a longer shelf life. Eating fast foods contain this kind of fat, "trans-fat", can lead to weight and fat gain in a short time.

Fast and junk foods also contain food additives or taste enhancers. There's an ingredient present in any fast food which is a type of salt called Ajinomoto. Chemically, it is called Monosodium Glutamate or MSG. Research studies have revealed that MSG is an Excitotoxin. According to Dr. Russell L. Blaylock and other researchers and medical journals, these are substances that damage the cells in the brain called the Neurons. As a result, they die. Unfortunately, there is no mechanism in humans that can separate this toxin from the blood and stop it from entering the brain. The region of the brain affected by this is called Hypothalamus. The damage caused to this section of the brain leads to abnormalities in the body. One such abnormality is Obesity. Many research studies, including that conducted by Russell L. Blaylock, M.D, has confirmed that the main reason for childhood obesity in the United States is the early exposure of children to Excitotoxin rich food products. Some of the other complications associated with early exposure to MSG are sleeping difficulties, impaired growth and emotional problems.

According to Dr. David Ludwig, the director of the obesity program at the children's hospital Boston, there is a close relation between fast food restaurants and obesity. Almost 1/3rd of the children in the United States eat fast food regularly. This increases the risk of obesity in children. The numbers are increasing at an alarming rate and it's hardly surprising as millions of dollars are spent on fast food advertising. Those advertisements know exactly how to make it almost impossible for people to avoid or ignore their products, especially children.

The following list of foods isn't the whole list of fast and junk foods, but just to give you an idea about some of the major foods that contribute to obesity and other health problems. Notice the common ingredients in these food items - have a high amount of calories, fat, trans-fat, carbohydrates, sodium (salt) and sugar. These ingredients are very tempting and addictive for children as well as adults.

Doughnuts: basically are deep fried, packed fully with sugar and fats. An average doughnut contains around 400 calories (1675 kJ) and other nutrients besides fat. According to many nutritionists and experts, eating lots of refined sugars add more sugar fluctuations to the blood.

Fried chicken and chicken nuggets: a single serving contains almost 420 calories (1760 kJ). It is also rich in sodium and saturated fat. Researches show that food cooked in highly heated oils can cause weight gain, cancer and other serious health problems.

Cheeseburger with French fries: this meal is packed with a lot of saturated fats. Saturated fats are found to contribute to strokes, heart attacks and a few types of cancers. A regular known brand of cheeseburger contains about 300 calories (1260 kJ) and around 240 calories (1005 kJ) are present in one serving of French fries topping around 540 calories (2260 kJ) and that's without a beverage. The approximate calories per serving in a cheese burger, fries with sauces, flavors and a drink, is somewhere between 600 - 1500 calories (2512-6280 kJ). That a whole day worth of calories can come from a single cheese burger meal. Health and medical experts say that beside the saturated fats and calories, cheeseburgers are a rich source of artery-clogging bad LDL cholesterol, sodium and trans-fat. Sodium causes water retention and can lead to weight gain and other blood pressure problems.

French Fries: usually every meal you buy from a fast food place comes with French fries. A cheese burger and a soda can have as many calories as two days' worth of food. French Fries are deep fried sticks of potatoes. They are loaded with trans-fats, saturated fats and sodium, which makes them high in artery-clogging fats. On the other hand, potatoes are rich in starch - which is simple carbohydrates. They are easily broken down into sugars. If we do not use up the energy readily provided by these sugars, then they are stored in the body as fat.

Pizza: the dough used in the crust itself is made of white flour, full of starch, simple carbohydrates, sugar, gluten and who knows what sort of yeast is used to make the pizza base or dough. Pizza is high in calories, fat and carbohydrate count. Topped with cheap full cream milk cheese and fattening processed meat toppings such as pepperoni, bacon and sausage. A slice of that pie could be well worth 600 calories (2512 kJ). Have two slices and you have exhausted your day worth of calories.

Hot dog: usually made of beef frank or sausage which is served in a sliced bun. Despite the bad nutrition in the sauces served with the meal, 80% of a hot dog is bad saturated fat. It contains sodium nitrite, a chemical salt used as a preservative and flavor enhancer in the franks. Researchers have claimed, nitrites could be carcinogenic (substance/s radionuclide or radiation which is an agent directly involved in causing cancers). Processed franks have a nutritional profile that will definitely raise the risks of heart disease and colon cancers.

Soda and drink: your beverage may contain large numbers of calories. For example, a large soda of 32 ounces (just below a liter or the big soda cup served with the big meal) gives you about 400 calories (1675 kJ). More about soda and measurements are in the "sugar the sweet toxin" chapter.

Processed meats: meats and their risks are not excluded from this small list. Sausages, hot dogs, bacon, jerky, packaged ham, pepperoni, salami and practically all red meat and lunch meats are categorized as processed - junk and fast foods because they are usually prepared with a carcinogenic ingredient known as sodium nitrite. This is used as a color fixer by meat companies to turn packaged meats into a bright red color so they appear fresh. According to the National Toxicology Program, Department of Health and Human Services, sodium nitrite also results in the formation of cancer-causing nitrosamines in the human body. This leads to a sharp increase in cancer risk for those who eat them. Sodium nitrate in processed meats is added as a preservative! There will be a whole chapter about meat later.

Another thing worth mentioning about meat is the poisoning gas pumped into the packaging. The United States Department of Agriculture (USDA) requires a seal to prove the meat has been inspected by a federal agency. However, that doesn't stop manufactures to inject Carbone Monoxide gas into the packaging. It's the same gas that comes out of your car exhaust pipe and it's pumped into the packaging of chicken, beef, pork, and fish. This practice is industry wide giving the meat the freshly cut look even after it's spoiled. Once the meat gets exposed to air it gradually turns brown or grey within just few day. But when Carbone Monoxide is pumped into the pre-packaged meat will keep it freshly looking even for weeks. Around 70% of meat purchased from your local supermarket are pumped with the colorless and odorless gas.

In 2002 the Food and Drug Administration (FDA) gave this practice a Generally Regarded As Safe (GRAS) status, and in 2004 the FDA approved this practice as a primary packaging method. The meat industry and whoever practices this are act backing this practice because they claim that consumers won't buy brown meat even if the meat is fresh and still well in time within its shelf-life. Despite the obvious health risk of long-term ingestion of Carbone Monoxide gas companies keep this practice to keep the cost of meat production low and deceive the consumer into buying meat pumped with poisonous gas and care less about the consumers' health outcome.

Other canned foods and soups: these are promoted as healthy foods but they are found to have high levels of artificial preservatives such as MSG, sodium and trans-fats as well as BPA which will be explained in details in the chapter "The Plastic Age".

Calories in fast foods: this list below will show you the amount of calories that most fast foods contain. These numbers aren't based on a particular brand but based on the most popular brands in the fast foods industry.

Fast Food Item	Amount	Calories/Kilojoules
Cheeseburger	Large	610 (2555 kJ)
Cheeseburger	Regular	320 (1340 kJ)
Hamburger	Large	520 (2177 kJ)
Hamburger	Regular	275 (1152 kJ)

Fish, Battered/Fried	1 serving	210 (876 kJ)
Chicken, Fried, Dark Meat	2 pieces	430 (1800 kJ)
Chicken, Fried, Wing/Breast	2 pieces	495 (2073 kJ)
Chicken Nuggets,	Plain 6	300 (1256 kJ)
Sausage, Fried/Battered	1	100 (418 kJ)
Onion Rings	8	175 (732 kJ)
Fries	Large	360 (1507)
Fries	Regular	240 (1005 kJ)
Hash Browns	1/2 cup	150 (628 kJ)
Corn Dog	1	460 (1926 kJ)
Hot Dog	Regular	240 (1005 kJ)
Hot Dog with Chili	1	325 (1360 kJ)
Dressing – Caesar	1 pkt	160 (670 kJ)
Dressing – French	1 pkt	160 (670 kJ)
Dressing – Ranch	1 pkt	230 (963 kJ)
Pancakes, Butter & Syrup	3	520 (2177 kJ)
Desserts – Brownie	1	245 (1025 kJ)
Desserts – Sundae, Caramel	1	305 (1277 kJ)

Desserts – Sundae, Hot Fudge	1	290 (1214 kJ)
Desserts – Sundae, Strawberry	1	270 (1130 kJ)
Desserts – Apple Pie	1	260 (1088 kJ)
Shakes – Chocolate	Regular	360 (1507 kJ)
Shakes – Strawberry	Regular	360 (1507 kJ)
Shakes – Vanilla	Regular	360 (1507 kJ)

Junk foods and premature death

According to the Federation of American Societies for Experimental Biology FASEB Journal, high levels of phosphates, which are mostly found in sodas and processed foods, accelerate signs of aging and high phosphate levels may also increase the prevalence and severity of age-related complications, such as chronic kidney disease and cardiovascular calcification, and can also induce severe muscle and skin atrophy.

M. Shawkat Razzaque, M.D., Ph.D., from the Department of Medicine, Infection and Immunity at the Harvard School of Dental Medicine, states, after examining the effects of high phosphate levels in mice, the results showed that phosphates have toxic effects, and may have a similar effect on other mammals, including humans. Dr. Razzaque said, "Humans need a healthy diet and keeping the balance of phosphate in the diet may be important for a healthy life and longevity". He also said: "Avoid phosphate toxicity and enjoy a healthy life."

Also, Gerald Weissmann, M.D., Editor-in-Chief of the FASEB Journal, says, "Soda is the caffeine delivery vehicle of choice for millions of people worldwide, but comes with phosphorus as a passenger". Dr. Weissmann also said in regard to the research "This research suggests that our phosphorus balance influences the ageing process, so don't tip it."

The US Department of Health and Human Services found combining a poor diet and a lack of physical activity cause 310,000 - 580,000 deaths every year. That's higher than deaths caused by guns or drug use. The types of foods that lead to death are ones with too much-saturated fat, trans-fat, sugar and sodium (salt) - which are all considered as fast foods and junk foods. Fast food meals often lack the nutrition the body needs such as whole grains, fruits and vegetables. This kind of diet leads to obesity, high blood pressure, diabetes, heart disease, stroke and cancers.

Fast foods and diabetes

According to the World Health Organization (WHO), diabetes is a group of metabolic diseases in which there are high blood sugar levels over a prolonged period. This high blood sugar produces the symptoms of frequent urination, increased thirst, and increased hunger. Also, diabetes occurs when the cells of the body are not able to take up sugar in the form of glucose. As a consequence, the amount of glucose in the blood is higher than normal. Over time, this raises the risk of heart disease and stroke, and can also cause damage to the kidneys, nerves and retinas. High blood glucose and diabetes are responsible for over five million deaths worldwide each year.

The world population in 2013 is estimated at 7.176 billion by the United States Census Bureau (USCB). However, 347 million adults in the world have diabetes, based on statistics in 2008, the analysis is published online by Lancet. While another more recent statistics released by the International Diabetes Federation (IDF), show in 2013, 387 million people worldwide live with diabetes, and this will reach 592 million people in the year 2035. That means almost every 6 seconds a person dies from diabetes or its related complications and in that same 6 seconds, 2 people will develop diabetes. It's estimated that 6.8% of all deaths worldwide are related to diabetes and its complications - which is around 5 million people every single year.

Those numbers are only for adults aged between 20 – 79 years. While children aged between 0 – 14 from a global population of 1.9 billion children under the age of 15, it's estimated that some 480,000 children in the world live with diabetes. This study estimates that annually around 76,000 children will develop Type 1 diabetes and the overall rate of increase is 3% worldwide. The greatest increase in new cases is in the age group under 5 years old, and many of them were born with diabetes.

Those numbers CANNOT be ignored. The latest research published by the American Heart Association's journal Circulation, found, people who consume fast food two or more times a week were found to increase the risk of developing Type 2 diabetes by 27%.

The effect of diabetes on the economy - The disaster with diabetes doesn't end with the health and the risks of people but it also affects the national and the international economy. For example, according to the American Diabetes Association, the total economic cost of diagnosed diabetes in 2012 is $245 billion, while there is a 41% increase from the previous estimate of $174 billion in the year 2007. (U.S population was 318,389,000 according to U.S. Census Bureau).

In the U.K, according to the National Health Service (NIH), a total estimation of £16 billion pounds is spent every year on treating diabetes and its complications. That means the NHS is spending over £1.8 million pounds in an hour or 11% of the NHS budget for England and Wales. This equates to over £30,000 pounds being spent on diabetes every minute. (UK population in 2015 was 65,110,00 according to Office for National Statistics).

According to the Australian Bureau of Statistics, Australia, with a population of 23,558,900 in 2014, the total annual cost for Australians with type 2 diabetes, is up to $6 billion annually based on the statistics of The Australian Diabetes, Obesity and Lifestyle study (AusDiab).

On the global scale, these statistics are based on the International Diabetes Federation (IDF):

Africa: In 2013 more than 20 million adults in Africa were estimated to have diabetes. That is 4.8% of Africans and only USD 4 billion was spent on treating diabetes in Africa in 2013.

Europe: 56 million adults living with diabetes - 8.5% Europeans. Diabetes caused 619,000 deaths across Europe in 2013. A total of 147 billion USD in 2013 spent on diabetes, which is more than 1 out of every 4 dollars spent on diabetes healthcare in the world was spent in this region.

The Middle East and North Africa (MENA): 1 in 10 adults in the Middle East and North Africa (MENA) region has diabetes, 35 million adults are currently living with diabetes in (MENA), 368,000 deaths related to diabetes in the region in 2013 and a total of only USD 13.6 billion was spent on diabetes healthcare in 2013.

America and Caribbean (NAC): More than 36 million people or 11% of adults in the North America and Caribbean (NAC) Region have diabetes. Diabetes caused 293,000 deaths in (NAC) in 2013 and this region spends the most healthcare dollars on diabetes in the whole world.

South and Central America (SACA): 24 million people with diabetes live in South and Central America (SACA) the equivalent of 8.0% of all adults in the Region or 1 adult in 12. In 2013 diabetes caused 226,000 deaths across the (SACA) region and 4.8% (USD 26.2 billion) of the global total of healthcare dollars devoted to diabetes were spent in this region.

South East Asia (SEA): Diabetes is a horrific threat in the South East Asia (SEA) Region. 72 million people with diabetes lived in South East Asia in 2013 that's one fifth of all adults with diabetes. In less than 20 years there will be 123 million people with diabetes according to the International Diabetes Federation (IDF) this is the South East Asian's real nightmare. The IDF also stated that despite the large numbers of people with diabetes across South East Asia, healthcare expenditures due to diabetes are estimated to have been only USD 6 billion (accounting for less than 1% of the global total) in 2013.

The Western Pacific (WP): 138 million people live with diabetes in the Western Pacific (WP) which is 8% of adults in 2013. 7 of the top 10 countries for diabetes prevalence are Pacific Islands. In 2013 diabetes caused 1.9 million deaths across the Western Pacific. The (WP) Region has the highest number of diabetes of all the IDF Regions. China alone had 1.3 million deaths due to diabetes in 2013.

World Facts: 382 million people had diabetes in 2013; by 2035 this will have risen to 592 million. 80% of people with diabetes live in low- and middle-income countries, 175 million people with diabetes are undiagnosed, and diabetes caused 5.1 million deaths worldwide in only 2013. Every six seconds, someone dies from diabetes-related complications, diabetes caused minimum USD $548 billion dollars in healthcare expenditures in 2013, 79,000 children developed type 1 diabetes in 2013 and more than 21 million live births were affected by diabetes during pregnancy in 2013 (from diabetic parent/s).

Despite the fact that it's around USD 550 billion printing money machine for the pharmaceutical industry in 2013 (that's more half a Trillion Dollar) and increasing. 400,000,000 million (400 billion) diabetic + 175,000,000 (175 million) are undiagnosed people living with diabetes in 2013. More than 5,000,000 (5 million) deaths in 2013 caused ONLY by diabetes and the numbers are growing. Think about it in any way suits you. It can be a conspiracy theory/fact and a designed world depopulation plan, or a disease with a hidden cure for profit orchestrated by the corporate elites or however way you want to digest it. The fact still remains, the next time you feed yourself or your family a junk meal, remember that everything comes at a price and this bill is a very expensive one.

Junk foods and heart disease

Junk foods contain low amounts of nutrition and high amounts of sodium, sweeteners, saturated and trans-fats, which can increase the risks of heart disease.

According to a study by researchers at McMaster University in Ontario, Canada, that included 52 countries, showed people who ate a "Western" diet based on meat, eggs and junk food were more likely to have heart attacks, while those who ate more fruits and vegetables had a lower risk. The research adds to the growing evidence that junk foods and animal fats can cause heart disease, in particular, heart attacks.

Also, according to a report from the workshop convened by the World Heart Federation, eating junk foods that contain saturated or trans fats may increase your blood levels of total and low-density lipoprotein cholesterol (which is the "bad" cholesterol) and decrease the blood levels of high-density lipoprotein cholesterol (the "good" cholesterol). Eating high amounts of trans-fats contributes to the risk of coronary heart disease, atherosclerosis, heart failure and cardiovascular hypertension.

Junk foods and liver diseases

Fast food diets can be highly toxic to the liver and other internal organs, as a recent study from Europe showed, an eating diet high in fat and sugar such as fast and junk foods could cause serious damage to the liver. Adding to the existed long list of health problems caused by junk foods, doctors have found fatty diets with levels of fructose similar to what is present in high fructose corn syrup (HFCS) can contribute to fatty liver disease. The findings are mostly significant to the increasing prevalence of fats and HFCS in our diets. It has been estimated that fructose accounts for nearly 10.2% of the daily caloric intake of most Americans. Fatty liver disease results in the accumulation of fat in the liver and when it accumulates at high enough levels, it can cause inflammation and scarring. This can compromise the functioning of the liver and can lead to liver failure.

More about that can be found in the chapter "Sugar the sweet toxins".

Junk foods and depressions

According to a recent study conducted by scientists from the University of Las Palmas de Gran Canarias and the University of Granada, eating fast and junk foods has a direct link to depression. Many people don't know the difference between depression, clinical depression and feeling sad or sadness. However, to down size the list of these three types, let's take first the feeling sad or sadness out of the list by briefly explaining it. Sadness or feeling sad is only a temporary mood state caused by boredom, routine or a loss etc. Mood state can change or can be "lifted up" by watching a comedy movie, visiting a friend or simply by doing something cheerful. While depression and clinical depression is a medical condition and can be very serious if it gets to the level of clinical depression - where it can become psychotic and requires medicine prescribed by a psychiatrist.

The relation between junk food and depression - Throughout my study of psychology and human behavior, I have done a lot of research regarding addictions and the effect of addictions on people. As I mentioned in the previous chapter "why are we getting fatter" and later in "sugar the sweet toxins", that sugar and sweeteners are addictive. And when people are addicted to something such as tobacco, alcohol and drugs, they exhibit addictive behaviors during the craving. Sugar is not different than the previous three. If you crave sugar, that's an addiction. Moreover, when it comes to food, some people get addicted to eating, and some to food in general. But the depression may take place in getting addicted on junk food meals. Besides the additives, the sugar and sweeteners are what have been imprinted in their minds from marketing and other methods of anchor patterns, which will be explained more in the following chapter "The media and the psychological factor".

Research shows, protein and amino acids in protein-rich foods such as fish, lean meats, eggs and legumes are the building blocks for many "happy" chemicals in the brain and their absence may cause a symptom of depression. Also, eating plenty of fresh vegetables, fruits, and whole grains decreases the risk of depression.

Nutritional doctors NDs advise eating healthy fats such as salmon, avocado, olive oil, and nuts because they are loaded with good natural fats. Unlike synthetic trans-fats which are widely found in many processed and junk foods. They also advise getting vitamins B (all chain of vitamins B), Folic acid, Omega 3, vitamin B6, and vitamin B12 as they all play a role in maintaining a healthy mood. Black-eyed peas, broccoli, shellfish, tuna, lamb, lean beef, and yoghurt are all rich sources of B vitamins.

More about this subject will be covered in the suggestions chapter.

Arthritis and joint disorders with fast and junk foods

By now, you already know that junk foods can cause weight-gain and obesity. Junk foods also cause diabetes type 1 & 2, increase the risk of heart disease and other health issues which will eventually lead to death. Furthermore, junk foods can also potentially cause osteoporosis (bone disease weakens the bones which may lead to bone's fracture).

According to a research by Ron Zernicke, the University of Michigan's School of Kinesiology, and C.Y Frank of the Alberta Bone at the Joint Health Institution, their research shows, excess sugar and fat in the body could weaken the bones and lead to osteoporosis, an ailment characterized by brittle bones. High saturated fat and sugar intake can stop calcium absorption which is what our bones need. Zernicke said "Right now, roughly 12 million Americans aged over 50 have osteoporosis" and "Baby Boomers, the oldest now 66, have reached the stage in life when they're most susceptible to bone and joint disorders."

Also, Linda K. Massey Ph.D. RD of Washington State University says that "sugar and fat aren't the only problems, but table salt, used in excess in the average diet, causes calcium loss". For every single teaspoon of salt consumed - 40 mg of calcium is lost through urine. Junk and fast foods contain lots of sodium in them. Also, salt can be addictive! Dr. Massey also added that "caffeine, salt, sugar, and saturated fat, these four bone breakers are the four basic food groups of the Standard American Diet (SAD)". If you're wondering about what food would contain caffeine, salt and sugar at the same time?! Well, all energy and sports drinks contain those three ingredients as well as any soda drink! You combine the four "bone breakers" when you drink soda with the high fat, saturated and trans-fat junk meal.

Junk food causes fatigue

Often when you eat fast and junk foods, you feel lazy and sometimes you just want to go to sleep. Although, it should be the other way around, because good fat gives you energy, unlike synthetic based fats such as trans-fats and saturated fats. Saturated fats are usually found in meats, mainly in burger meat, chicken, bacon, beef, sausage and ham. It can be also found in cheese, butter and margarine. On the other hand, trans-fats are primarily found in fats being used to fry fast foods, especially at fast food restaurants. These include French fries, breaded or crumbed fish, onion rings, French toast sticks etc. They are also found in pre-packed or pre-half fried junk foods before packing, such as frozen fries, frozen pizzas and canned food.

Saturated fats are a challenge for the body to digest. Digesting saturated fats requires diversion of blood and oxygen to the digestive system leading to over-work the organs and muscles which can produce fatigue. The body spends a tremendous amount of energy on digesting such difficult fats as saturated fats, while at the same time taking care of the rest of the organs by providing blood and oxygen, especially to the brain. Therefore, it will be overwhelming for the body to do all that at once. Hence, the brain will send a message to the body to do fewer activities, especially physical work that require muscle activities to work less in order to burn the bad fats and recover. I once had a client who participated in a burger eating competition, which landed him in a coma. This was mainly due to the large amount of saturated and trans-fats he consumed!

Junk food causes stroke

According to a study at the University of California San Francisco, people who are highly stressed and eat a diet rich in fat and sugar are at an increased risk of developing health problems, as opposed to lower stressed people with a similar diet chart.

Kirstin Aschbacher, PhD, an assistant professor in the UCSF Department of Psychiatry and lead author stated in a statement "Many people think a calorie is a calorie, but this study suggests that two women who eat the same thing could have different metabolic responses based on their level of stress." Also, "There appears to be a stress pathway that works through diet - for example, it could be similar to what we see in animals, where fat cells grow faster in response to junk food when the body is chronically stressed."

The body can be heavily stressed when it tries to do many things at once, especially if it is something not easily registered by the brain. The brain then will have no choice but to give an order to the body to shut down partially, (as a stroke), or fully, (as in coma) and permanently as death (if the body runs out of energy due to heavy stress). Think of a computer, when you open too many internet pages, the computer is already stressed in keeping the anti-virus in operation. Then you open music and video files at once, your computer will freeze, sometimes shuts down. If the computer was hit with a virus while already heavily stressed, the computer will just die and become part of history. A similar concept can be applied to our physiology and the relation between stroke and junk foods. These junk foods such as candy and other sweets, fried snacks, soda drinks and some fast-food products all contribute to cardiovascular risks by upsetting the nutritional balance in your diet. When you eat more fat and sugar than fiber, vitamins and minerals you might develop weight and arterial problems. These conditions increase the risks of potentially fatal heart attack, stroke and related complications.

Gallbladder disease and junk foods

The gallbladder is a small hollow organ that sits beneath the right lobe of the liver. The Gallbladder stores bile for the liver before it is released into the small intestine. Bile is a dark green to yellowish brown fluid produced by the liver to help the digestion of fats and in breaking down the fats in the small intestine. A gallbladder attack can occur as a result of a gallstone blocking the ducts that connect the gallbladder to the liver. This can lead to sharp and intense pain. Fast and junk foods can trigger gallbladder attacks because of the high amounts of fat found in most junk foods - which are difficult for the body to break down. A gallbladder attack can lead to surgery to remove the gallbladder.

Cancers and junk foods

Cancer is the modern nightmare of humanity, it's the blind grim reaper who doesn't differentiate between male and female, age and race, rich and poor and even animals. Many people were and will be prey to cancer. If we can't do anything about it, then at least we can educate ourselves and others about it. Learning about it will help us to be in a position to prevent it and keep it at bay. As I always say to my clients and students "knowing your challenge is the first half of your victory". I am a big believer in education, knowledge and research. Nothing can change, develop, evolve and be perfected without knowledge and will.

Just to be fair and clear, foods and junk/fast foods are not alone in causing cancers. They are just one reason of many out there, like alcohol, tobacco, obesity, as well as an unhealthy lifestyle. There are many factors playing a big role in the development of cancer/s in our modern days such as chemicals, infections and diseases. The exposure to radiation is also a reason and we're being bombarded with radiation almost all the time and everywhere even in our own homes, such as the electrical/phone poles next to our homes, cellphones, Wi-Fi modems and other electronic devices are emitting radiation constantly. Moreover, beside the stated factors in causing cancers, cancers are also heredity (inherited genetically) and can be related to hormones and other pathogenic factors such as genetics, epigenetics, metastasis (tumors). In this book and especially in this segment I'll be focusing more on the effect of diet and foods on cancers. Also, from time to time I might include some researches related to the subject which I have found during my research and while I was writing this book.

According to Dietitians Association of Australia, the foods we eat in general contain numerous amounts of nutrients and chemicals. Many of them can protect and prevent us against cancers, while some others can increase the risk of cancers. There are more than 100 types of cancers according to the National Cancer Institute. To determine how diet can affect the risks of cancers or accelerate cancer risks would be an extremely complicated task since every individual has a different type of diet. And the effect of a diet may vary from one person to another.

However, some studies show that there are certain foods can assist in accelerating the risks of cancers.

Arsenic and cancers related to junk foods

According to recent studies, there is a lot of arsenic in rice krispies, rice-cake and crackers. These products are many children favorite breakfast and adult's snacks choice. Rice is rich in protein, fiber and vitamins but also it's the only common food item with high levels of arsenic. Although, arsenic is a naturally occurring element found in the environment. Many companies have labs made of inorganic arsenic to pesticide, and rice easily observes it in high levels. According to the Agency for Toxic Substances and Disease, regular exposure to small amounts of arsenic can increase the risk of bladder, lung and skin cancer as well as type two diabetes. Children are at a higher risk because since they weigh less and they are exposed to more arsenic per pound or Kg. Often, one serve of rice for a child is over the weakly recommended arsenic limits. Rice cereal, rice cakes, rice crackers, rice treats and sweets they all include significant levels of inorganic arsenic that can be harmful.

Genetically modified organisms (GMOs):

As stated in a previous chapter, according to the World Health Organization (WHO), genetically modified organisms (GMOs) are "organisms in which the genetic material (DNA) has been altered in such a way that it does not occur naturally." Our DNA has been written and harmoniously coded by nature, the environment as well as or diet including plants and animals. Since our DNA has been evolved by nature and took thousands or millions of years to evolve - as well as an incredible immune system to protect us from other viruses, diseases and bacterial threats – then, how do you think our DNA will react and deal with new synthetic genes?

If the DNA of an organism has been enhanced, altered or changed at the genetic level and been placed into the food and animals which we consume, don't you think that would eventually affect us? How about the plants and animals which are also part of our diets - they have also been genetically altered - wouldn't it be absurd to ignore millions of years of evolution and think altering/changing genetic codes will not back-fire on us and the environment? There is a price of everything and it will be paid by a law called "Cause and Effect". We caused it and we'll pay for it.

More about that can be found in a previous chapter "GMO/GE food V.S organic food" Segment "Are GMOs dangerous? And do GMOs cause cancer?"

Processed meats

The majority of processed meat products including lunch meats, bacon, sausage, hot dogs etc., contain chemical preservatives that make them appear fresh and appealing. Although they may draw the buyer in, they also can be a cause of cancer. It's common that sodium nitrate has been linked to significantly increasing the risk of colon and other forms of cancer.

Microwaved food

This is still controversial - some scientists claim that microwave ovens may leave some radiation residuals in the foods, and many another claim that the amount of residuals left aren't enough to cause any type of cancer. Also, according to cancer research centers such as Cancer Research UK, "Microwave ovens don't make foods radioactive. They just heat them. Microwave ovens heat food by producing radiation which is absorbed by water molecules in the food. This makes the water molecules vibrate and produce heat, which cooks the food". Some argue about the radiation which is absorbed by the water molecules in the food as this absorbed radiation stays in the water molecules which we then consume. However, this is still controversial, but many studies indicate that it is not enough to cause cancer, and microwave ovens are safe to use if you follow the instructions of use.

Pancreatic cancer linked to soda and soft drinks

The pancreas lies behind the stomach, it makes hormones such as insulin to balance the sugar level in the blood and produces juices with enzymes to help break down fats and protein in foods.

Sadly many people admit to drinking more soda than water each day, and sometimes no water at all. Soda drinks aren't only bad because of the high amount of sugar they contain or because of leading the nation to obesity, (as studies and facts have provided regarding the risks of sugar, high sugar corn syrup HFCS and other sweeteners in the chapter "sugar the sweet toxin"). There are many alarming studies indicating serious risks with soda drinks as eventually may lead to cancer.

A study lead by author Noel T. Mueller, MPH, a research associate at the Cancer Control Program at Georgetown University Medical Center, Washington, D.C. The study is published in Cancer Epidemiology, Biomarkers & Prevention, a journal of the American Association for Cancer Research. He stated that "People who drank two or more soft drinks a week had an 87% increased risk or nearly twice the risk of pancreatic cancer compared to individuals consuming no soft drinks"

The reaction from the multi-billion dollar beverage industry was as expected. They denied and doubted the legitimacy of the study by calling it "flawed", and also pointed to other research that has found no association between soda consumption and pancreatic cancer.

Furthermore, according to American Cancer Society, cancer of the pancreas was diagnosed in about 42,000 people in the U.S. in 2009, and estimates about 35,240 deaths from the disease were expected.

Previous studies have shown mixed conclusions regarding the consumption of soft drinks and the increases in the risk of pancreatic cancer. The study by Muller and his colleagues involved 60,524 men and women enrolled in the Singapore Chinese Health Study. It began in 1993 and lasted up to 14 years, looking at their diet if they got cancer. They asked all participants about food intake, including sodas and juices. Mueller said "the researchers didn't ask specifically about diet soda consumption", but noted that most of the soda drinks were regular or sweetened. In Singapore at that time, Mueller said: "there was very little intake of diet soda". However, they found 140 cases of pancreatic cancer and looked back to see if there was an association with sodas or juices.

The research was done as follow - they divided the consumption of sodas and juices into three categories: none, less than two servings a week and two or more servings a week. The group that drank two or more a week - the average number was five, had 87% increased risk. Muller said, "No link was found between juices and pancreatic cancer risk."

Moreover, the link with sugary sodas is, as Mueller said "What we believe is the sugar in the soft drinks is increasing the insulin level in the body, which we think contributes to pancreatic cancer cell growth. That increase in insulin is what may be leading to the development of cancer." Mueller's team adjusted for other risk factors such as advancing age, smoking, diabetes, and body mass index. The risk for pancreatic cancer rises with age.

Soda drinks have a unique color especially the dark-brown cola. They are usually made with what the beverage industry calls a "caramel" color. Whether that brown color resembles caramel or black water to you, it doesn't change the fact that this color is added artificially to make the drink look more appealing to consumers. Many people never thought about it or even wondered if this color contains any harmful substances or has any risks related to it. The coloring substances used in cola drinks brands is a potentially carcinogenic chemical called 4-methylimidazole (4-Mel).

According to the Office of Environmental Health Hazards Assessment (OEHHA) which is a specialized department within the cabinet-level of California Environmental Protection Agency (Cal/EPA) (with responsibility for assessing and evaluating health risks from environmental chemical contaminants), OEHHA states that 4-methylimidazole (4-Mel) which is used in beverages for coloring, "4-Methylimidazole (4-MEI) is a compound used to make certain pharmaceuticals, photographic chemicals, dyes and pigments, cleaning and agricultural chemicals and rubber products.

4-MEI is formed during the production of certain caramel coloring agents used in many foods and drink products. It may also be formed during the cooking, roasting, or other processing of some foods and beverages." People are usually consuming (4-Mel) in their foods and beverages and there are many products that potentially contain 4-MEI including certain colas, beers, soy sauces, bread, coffee, etc.

Also, the same report states, regarding the dangers and health risks that may occur in being exposed to 4-methylimidazole (4-Mel), the reports say "Studies published in 2007 by the federal government's National Toxicology Program showed that long-term exposure to 4-MEI resulted in increases in lung's cancer in male and female mice. These findings were the basis for the addition of 4-MEI to California's Proposition 65 list of carcinogens. Exposure to high concentrations of 4-MEI (such as concentrations that might occur in industrial settings) is reported to irritate the lungs or burn the eyes and skin."

Furthermore, on January 7, 2012, under California's Proposition 65 law, any food or beverage sold in the state of California that exposes consumers to more than 29 micrograms of 4-Mel per day is supposed to carry a health-warning label. Also, the manufacturers were required to label a product sold in the state with a cancer warning if it exposes consumers to more than 29 micrograms of 4-Mel per day. The exposure comes from consumption.

The California Office of Environmental Health Hazard Assessment used 29 micrograms as a maximum limit based on the level they determined poses a one in 100,000 risks of cancer. Some private organizations have done their own tests on different soda drinks brands to see how much of 4-MEI each brand contains, and they found some 352.5 micrograms of 4-MEI per one can! The research and result can be easily found for public viewing.

Another study has been conducted in regards to soda and sweet beverages and their links to cancer by a team of researchers led by Maki Inoue-Choi, PhD, MS, RD, a research associate in the Division of Epidemiology and Community Health of the University Of Minnesota School Of Public Health in Minneapolis. The study has found, postmenopausal women who consumed sugar-sweetened beverages were at a greater risk of developing endometrial cancer than women who didn't consume sugary drinks. The study also indicated, the more sugar-based beverages they consumed, the higher their cancer risks.

Just a little brief of what is "endometrial cancer". According to Oxford Medical Journal, Endometrial cancer: ESMO Clinical Practice Guidelines for diagnosis, treatment and follow-up, endometrial cancers are divided into two categories; type I, which is driven by the female hormone oestrogen, and type 2, which is not dependent on oestrogen. Endometrial cancer is now the most common gynecological malignancy in Europe and North America, and according to the same medical journal regarding the causality of this cancer states "Risk factors for developing endometrial cancer are: obesity, nulliparity, late menopause, diabetes mellitus and prolonged, unopposed estrogen exposure, tamoxifen and the oral contraceptive pill." It seems almost all of these risk factors are inside that can of soda!

Going back to Dr. Maki Inoue-Choi's research, it confirms that endometrial cancer is associated with anything increases oestrogen levels and obesity in women. Dr. Inoue-Choi says "Other studies have shown increasing consumption of sugar-sweetened beverages has paralleled the increase in obesity. Obese women tend to have higher levels of oestrogens and insulin than women of normal weight. Increased levels of oestrogens and insulin are established risk factors for endometrial cancer." The study and many others show clearly the dangers and risks that can be caused by high amounts of sweet sugars in soda beverages, and the devastating results which can lead to obesity - and obesity leads to hormonal imbalances, cancers and deaths.

Soda and sweet beverages are contained in cans as well as plastic bottles which add more risks to our health as well the environment. More studies regarding the risk of sweeteners such as HFCS, Aspartame and sugar will be in the chapter "sugar the sweet toxin" and also the relation between plastic and cancer can be found in the chapter on "The Plastic Age".

Bad carbohydrates and the link to cancers

As we know by now from the chapter "why we're getting fat" subheading "understanding carbohydrates", there are good carbs and bad carbs. Carbohydrates can turn into fat, and fat leads to obesity if you consume more carbohydrates than you burn. Those extra calories convert into fat and can be stored in the body. The conversion of excess carbohydrates to fat is a complex process and occurs primarily when you frequently consume too many calories per day.

However, is there any link between carbs and cancer? Well, a journal published in 2011 by Dr. Klement and Dr. Kämmerer, Duke University in Durham, North Carolina, published a comprehensive review of the literature involving dietary carbohydrates and their direct and indirect effect on cancer cells. The study was published in the journal, Nutrition and Metabolism and can be found on the National Center for Biotechnology Information, U.S. National Library of Medicine website under article information "Is there a role for carbohydrate restriction in the treatment and prevention of cancer?" It's a very interesting article, Dr. Klement and Dr. Kämmerer hypothesized that by reducing the amount of dietary carbohydrates, one could suppress or delay the emergence of cancer and/or the proliferation of tumor cells already present.

Many scientists, practitioners and nutritionists have known this for years; Prof. Robert Lustig, the University of California, San Francisco has written and lectured about this also. They all hypothesize limiting carbohydrates could suppress or slow the growth of cancers.

According to Dr. Klement, "Cancer cells thrive on glucose and starve on fats and ketones, which are food-derived energy units that are plentiful in low-carbohydrate diets." Also According to Dr. Freedland (colleague of Dr. Klement), "The commonplace advice to avoid dietary fat is not a good recommendation to give cancer patients. They should eat a lot of fat and avoid sugar."

According to the Duke University, a study will involve calorie restriction in men with prostate cancer. Calorie restriction means cutting down on carbohydrates intake. The study has a projected end date of 2016, and it's being funded by the National Cancer Institute and the Atkins Foundation, which is a philanthropic outgrowth of the famous Atkins diet enterprise. The study will employ an Atkins-like diet, where carbohydrates are severely restricted to less than 20 grams a day.

Carbohydrates are one of the three macronutrients, the other two being fats and protein. And as stated in a previous chapter "why are we getting fat" subheading "understanding carbohydrates", there are simple carbohydrates and complex carbohydrates. Simple carbohydrates include sugars which are found naturally in foods such a fruits and fruit juices, sodas, some vegetables, white bread, white rice, pasta, milk and milk products, most snack foods, sweets, etc. But let us not forget the simple sugars added to foods during processing and refining are the "bad carbs". It's the simple sugars that get most of the credit for causing the insulin response and glycation-associated inflammation that can lead to cancer. Therefore, by reducing the amount of simple carbohydrates in the diet, the emergence of cancer can be suppressed or delayed, or the proliferation of already existing tumor cells can be slowed down, stopped, and reversed by depriving the cancer cells of the food they need for survival. Drs. Rainer Klement and Ulrike Kämmerer indicated this in the journal "Nutrition and Metabolism 2011".

Refined sugars and cancers

The same goes for refined sugars as refined carbohydrates, which also cause a rapid spike in insulin levels and feed the growth of cancer cells. Fructose-rich sweeteners like high-fructose corn syrup (HFCS) are particularly offensive, as cancer cells have been shown to quickly and easily metabolize them in order to proliferate. And since cookies, cakes, pies, sodas, juices, sauces, cereals, and many other popular, mostly processed, food items are loaded with HFCS and other refined sugars, this helps explain why cancer rates are on the rise these days.

Farmed salmon and its relation to cancer

According to Dr. David Carpenter, Director of the Institute for Health and the Environment at the University of Albany farmed salmon is another high-risk cancer food not only because of the lack of vitamin D, but it is often contaminated with carcinogenic chemicals, PCBs (polychlorinated biphenyls), flame retardants and pesticides.

Note, this doesn't apply on all salmon! It only applies on commercially farmed salmon.

Conclusion

Certainly, nothing good comes from junk and fast foods. As fast foods are deficient in fibers which are essential for proper digestion and help in preventing constipation and irregular bowel movements. There is no benefit from this kind of food whatsoever. The only beneficiary is the fast and junk food industry empire. This is while infesting the world with its junk and affecting people with all sorts of diseases and health issues, especially the poor, working and middle-class population.

"You are what you eat so don't be fast, cheap, easy or fake."

- Unknown

"Every living cell in your body is made from the food you eat. If you eat junk food you'll have a junk body."

- Jeanette Jenkins

Chapter 6
Processed Food

Processed foods have earned a bad reputation as a bad diet and nutritional source. Processed foods are directly linked to for obesity, high blood pressure, type 2 diabetes along with other illnesses and diseases. However, when a person is being asked about what is processed food the answers will vary from one person to another. Some people think of processed food is only packed and canned food. But the fact is, processed food is more than just boxed pizza, potato chips and drive-thru burgers. It may be a surprise to you to know that whole-wheat/grain bread; homemade soup, sauces, a chocolate bar and even a chopped apple in a bag or box sold at supermarkets are also processed foods.

What is the definition of processed food? In fact, in the context of food, the word "processed" is not legally defined yet. The International Food Information Council Foundation defines processed foods as "Any deliberate change in a food that occurs before it's available for us to eat." That means almost all kinds of foods that are available these days on supermarket shelves or at fancy restaurants and even cheap fast take-out foods are also considered "processed".

Here is a brief explanation of what processed food is capable of doing to us. According to the George Mateljan Foundation, indicating, the variety of additives included in processed foods are thought to have the ability to compromise the body's structure and functions and are also suggested to be related to the development of skin, pulmonary (serious lung disorder) and psycho-behavioral conditions. Also, Butylated hydroxytoluene (BHT) and butylated hydroxyanisole (BHA) are currently being investigated for their potentials to damage genetic materials and therefore, promote cancer. Sulfites have been found to aggravate asthma (hypertext) in certain children and adults. Artificial colorings have been noted to cause hypersensitivity reactions in sensitive persons promoting conditions such as ADHD (attention-deficit-hyperactivity disorder), asthma and skin conditions such as urticaria and atopic dermatitis (eczema). Therefore, the study encourages people to avoid processed foods that contain these and other chemical additives that may greatly contribute to health issues.

Processed foods additives

Food additives are substances added to foods to preserve flavor or enhance its taste and appearance. Some additives have been used for centuries; for example, preserving food by pickling (with vinegar), salting as with meat and fish, preserving sweets, or using sulfur dioxide in some wines. With the advent of processed foods in the second half of the 20th century, many more additives have been introduced, of both natural and artificial origins.

Nowadays food additives vary and can be divided into several groups. Although, there are some similarities between them and here is a list of the most widely used food additives and a brief elaboration about their purposes:

Acids: food acids are added to make flavors "sharper", and also act as preservatives and antioxidants. Common food acids include vinegar, citric acid, tartaric acid, malic acid, fumaric acid, and lactic acid.

Acidity regulators: are used to change or otherwise control the acidity and alkalinity of foods.

Anticaking agents keep powders such as milk powder from caking or sticking.

Antifoaming agents: reduce or prevent foaming in foods.

Antioxidants: such as vitamin C act as preservatives by inhibiting the effects of oxygen on food. This can be beneficial to health.

Bulking agents: such as starches are additives that increase the bulk of a food without affecting its taste.

Food coloring: these are added to food to replace colors lost during preparation, or/and to make food look more attractive.

Color retention agents: are used to preserve a food's existing color.

Emulsifiers: allow water and oils to remain mixed together in an emulsion, as in mayonnaise, ice cream, and homogenized milk.

Flavors: are additives that give food a particular taste or smell and may be derived from natural ingredients or created artificially.

Flavor enhancers: these enhance a food's existing flavors. They may be extracted from natural sources (through distillation, solvent extraction, maceration, among other methods) or created artificially.

Flour treatment agents: are added to flour to improve its color or its use in baking.

Glazing agents provide a shiny appearance or protective coating to foods.

Humectants: prevent foods from drying out.

Tracer gas allows for package integrity testing to prevent foods from being exposed to the atmosphere to guarantee a longer shelf life.

Preservatives: to prevent or inhibit spoilage of food due to the action of fungi, bacteria and other microorganisms.

Stabilizers: thickeners and gelling agents, such as agar or pectin (used in jams and similar products) give foods a firmer texture. While they are not true emulsifiers, they help to stabilize emulsions.

Sweeteners: are added to foods for flavoring. Sweeteners other than sugar are added to keep the food energy (calories) low, or because they have beneficial effects for people suffering from diabetes mellitus and tooth decay and diarrhea.

Thickeners are substances when added to the mixture, increase its viscosity without substantially modifying its other properties.

These are some of the major Food Additives which are used in processed foods. However, to regulate these additives and inform consumers, each additive is assigned a unique number, termed as "E numbers". The number is used in Europe for all approved additives. This numbering scheme has now been adopted and extended by the Codex Alimentarius Commission to internationally identify all additives regardless of whether they are approved for use or not.

E numbers are all prefixed by the letter "E". However, countries outside Europe use only the number, whether the additive is approved in Europe or not. For example, Acetic Acid is written as E260 on products sold in Europe but is simply known as additive 260 in some countries. Additive 103, alkanet, is not approved for use in Europe, so does not have an E number. Although, it is approved for use in Australia and New Zealand. Since 1987, Australia has had an approved system of labelling for additives in packaged foods. Each food additive has to be named or numbered. The numbers are the same as in Europe but without the prefix letter "E".

The United States Food and Drug Administration (FDA) lists these items as "Generally Recognized as Safe" (GRAS). They are listed under both their Chemical Abstracts Service number and FDA regulation under the United States Code of Federal Regulations.

The top 10 Food Additives to Avoid

Food additives have been used for centuries to enhance the appearance and flavor of foods and to extend their shelf-life. We know these food additives exist in our foods based on the studies and labeling. However, do these food additives really "add" any value or nutritional value to your food? If not, do they "add" any risk to our health and the environment, especially nowadays where food is owned and controlled by greedy food corporations?

Furthermore, the reason in adding food additives to our foods is to make it easier for the food industries to process, package and store the foods for the consumer. There's another valid question can also be raised in this regard - how do we know what kind of food additives is in a packet of pizza, a carton of milk or even in baby formulas? And why does it have such a long shelf-life (expiry date)? Also, if that food has preservative agents in it to keep it preserved for a longer life on the shelves, boxes, bags or packages, then what about if our bodies also preserve it (based on its preservative agents). When we consume it, it might also stay inside our bodies for a longer time before the body completely breaks it down and gets rid of it.

According to the United States Department of Agriculture Economic Research Services USDA, a typical American household spends about 90 percent of their food budget on processed foods because it's cheaper and easier to prepare. Also, not to forget that it's addictive (because of the amount of artificial sweeteners and other food agents in it). The exposure to a large amount of artificial food additives, many of which can cause dire consequences to their health, might not be cheap and easy after all.

Scientifically speaking, some food additives are worse than others. Here's a list of the top 10 food additives you're recommended to avoid and then I'll include some honorary mentions of other food additives to avoid, or in this case I should say "dishonorary mentions".

1. Artificial Sweeteners

Aspartame, (E951) more popularly known as NutraSweet® and Equal, is found in foods labelled "diet, light or sugar-free". Aspartame is believed to be carcinogenic and accounts for more adverse reactions than all other foods and food additives combined. Aspartame is not your friend. Aspartame is a neurotoxin and carcinogen. Known to erode intelligence and affect short-term memory, the components of this toxic sweetener may lead to a wide variety of ailments including brain tumor, diseases such as lymphoma, diabetes, multiple sclerosis, Parkinson's, Alzheimer's, fibromyalgia, and chronic fatigue. And also emotional disorders such depression and anxiety attacks, dizziness, headaches, nausea, mental confusion, migraines and seizures. Acesulfame-K, a relatively new artificial sweetener found in baking goods, gum and gelatin. It has not been thoroughly tested and has been linked to kidney tumors.

Found in - diet or sugar free sodas, zero and diet barrages, jelly (gelatins), desserts, sugar free gum, drink mixes, baking goods, table top sweeteners, cereal, breathmints, pudding, kool-aid, ice tea, chewable vitamins, toothpastes and others diet food products. More about Aspartame will be in the chapter "Sugar the sweet toxin".

2. High Fructose Corn Syrup

High fructose corn syrup (HFCS), is a highly-refined artificial sweetener which has become the number one source of calories in America and many other countries. It is found in almost all processed foods. HFCS packs on the weight faster than any other ingredient, increases your LDL (bad) cholesterol levels, and contributes to the development of diabetes and tissue damage, among other harmful effects.

Found in: most processed foods, breads, candy, flavored yoghurts, salad dressings, canned vegetables, cereals, beverages and others. More about HFCS will be in the chapter "Sugar the sweet toxin".

3. Monosodium Glutamate (MSG / E621)

MSG is an amino acid used as a flavor enhancer in soups, salad dressings, chips, frozen entrees, and many restaurant foods. MSG is known as an excitotoxin, a substance that overexcites cells to the point of damage or death. Studies show that regular consumption of MSG may result in adverse side effects including depression, disorientation, eye damage, fatigue, headaches, and obesity. MSG affects the neurological pathways of the brain and disconnects the "I'm full" function, which explains the effects of weight gain.

Found in: Many Asian restaurants, many snacks, chips, cookies, seasonings, most soup products, frozen dinners, lunch meats and others.

4. Trans-Fat

Trans-fat is used to enhance and extend the shelf life of food products and is among the most dangerous substances that you can consume. Found in deep-fried fast foods and certain processed foods made with margarine or partially hydrogenated vegetable oils. Trans-fats are formed by a process called hydrogenation. Numerous studies show that trans-fat increases LDL (bad cholesterol) levels while decreasing HDL (good cholesterol). This increases the risk of heart attacks, heart disease and strokes, and contributes to increased inflammation, diabetes and other health problems. Oils and fats are now forbidden on the Danish market if they contain trans-fatty acids exceeding 2 per cent, a move that effectively bans partially hydrogenated oils.

Found in: margarine, chips and crackers, baked goods, fast foods, fried foods, canned foods and others.

5. Common Food Dyes

Studies show, artificial coloring found in soda, fruit juices and salad dressings, may contribute to behavioral problems in children and lead to a significant reduction in IQ levels. Animal studies have linked other food coloring to cancer. The followings are highly considered to be avoided:

Blue #1 and Blue #2 (E133): banned in Norway, Finland and France. May cause chromosomal damage. - Found in: candy, cereal, soft drinks, sports drinks and pet foods

Red dye # 3 (also Red #40 – a more current dye) (E124): banned from use in many foods and cosmetics in 1990 after 8 years of debate. This dye continues to be on the market until supplies run out! Has been proven to cause thyroid cancer and chromosomal damage in laboratory animals, may also interfere with brain-nerve transmission. - Found in: fruit cocktail, maraschino cherries, cherry pie mix, ice cream, candy, bakery products and more!

Yellow #6 (E110) and Yellow Tartrazine (E102): banned in Norway and Sweden. Increases the number of kidney and adrenal gland tumors in laboratory animals, may cause chromosomal damage. - Found in: American cheese, macaroni and cheese, candy and carbonated beverages, lemonade and more...

6. Sodium Sulphite (E221)

The preservative used in wine-making and other processed foods. According to the FDA, approximately 1 in 100 people are sensitive to sulphites in foods. The majority of these individuals are asthmatic, suggesting a link between asthma and sulphites. Individuals who are sulphite sensitive may experience headaches, breathing problems, and rashes. In severe cases, sulphites can actually cause death by closing down the airway altogether, leading to cardiac arrest.

Found in: Wine and dried fruit

7. Sodium Nitrate/Sodium Nitrite

Sodium nitrate (or sodium nitrite) is used as a preservative, coloring and flavoring agent in bacon, ham, hotdogs, luncheon meats, corned beef, smoked fish and other processed meats. This ingredient sounds harmless, but it's actually highly carcinogenic once it enters the human digestive system. It forms a variety of nitrosamine compounds that enter the bloodstream and wreak havoc with a number of internal organs - the liver and pancreas in particular. Sodium nitrite is widely regarded as a toxic ingredient, and the USDA actually tried to ban this additive in the 1970's but was vetoed by food manufacturers who complained as they had no alternative for preserving packaged meat products. Why does the industry still use it? Simply and as I explained in the previous chapter, this chemical just happens to turn meats bright red. It's actually a color fixer, and it makes old, dead meats appear fresh and vibrant.

Found in: hotdogs, bacon, ham, luncheon meat, cured meats, corned beef, smoked fish or any other type of processed meat

8. BHA and BHT (E320)

Butylated hydroxyanisole (BHA) and butylated hydrozyttoluene (BHT) are preservatives found in cereals, chewing gum, potato chips, and vegetable oils. This common preservative keeps foods from changing color, changing flavor, or becoming rancid. It affects the neurological system of the brain, alters behavior and has potential to cause cancer. BHA and BHT are oxidants that form cancer-causing reactive compounds in the body. Found in: Potato chips, gum, cereal, frozen sausages, enriched rice, lard, shortening, candy, jelly (jello) and other children candies.

9. Sulphur Dioxide (E220)

Sulphur additives are toxic, and in the United States, the Federal and Drugs Administration FDA has prohibited their use on raw fruit and vegetables. Adverse reactions include bronchial problems particularly in those prone to asthma, hypotension (low blood pressure), flushing, tingling sensations or anaphylactic shock. It also destroys vitamins B1 and E. Not recommended for consumption by children. The International Labor Organization says to avoid E220 if you suffer from conjunctivitis (eye infection/s), bronchitis (inflammation airways), emphysema (lung disease that causes shortness of breath), bronchial asthma, or cardiovascular disease.

Found in: beer, soft drinks, dried fruit, juices, cordials, wine, vinegar, and potato products.

10. Potassium Bromate

An additive used to increase volume in some white flour, bread, and rolls. Potassium bromate is known to cause cancer in animals. Even small amounts in bread can create problems for humans.

Found in: bread

These are the top 10 food additives and highly recommended to avoid, especially for children. These implications are based on valid studies showing some significant and alarming results of negative side effects to avoid these food additives and coloring.

Furthermore, here are some dishonorary mentions of other food additives and also highly recommended to avoid:

The artificial colors in many cases are proven to cause hives and asthma in aspirin-sensitive asthmatics. And they were used to test children's bad behavior in the Southampton Study published on April 10, 2008.

Artificial Colors: 102, 107, 110, 122-129, 132, 133, 142, 151, 155, 160b (annatto)

Preservatives:

- Sorbates 200, 201, 202, 203
- Benzoates 210, 211, 212, 213
- Sulphites 220, 221, 222, 223, 224, 225, 226, 227, 228
- Nitrates, nitrites 249, 250, 252
- Propionates 280, 281, 282, 283
- Flavor Enhancers:
- Glutamates and MSG 620, 621, 622, 623, 624, 625
- Disodium guanylate 627
- Disodium inosinate 631
- Ribonucleotides 635
- Hydrolysed Vegetable Protein (HVP) – no number

FDA Generally Regarded As Safe (GRAS) and food additives

There's a process of additives, GMO and GE for foods called "GRAS" or Generally Regarded As Safe, in this process the FDA permits food manufactures do their own testing to decide independently whether ingredients are safe or not. Upon determining if the additive or GMO is GRAS or not the company can voluntarily submit its findings to the FDA. Voluntarily means, there are no industry-wide testing regulations for new food additives. Or, as FDA spokesperson Theresa Eisenman said, "It is the manufacturer's responsibility to ensure that the [GMO] food products it offers for sale are safe..." Companies have a significant degree of discretion of which ingredients they add without pre-mark it as FDA approval because they can make their own GRAS determination. Although, even when companies submit their data the FDA does not see the complete data and studies is a problem.

According to a Biotechnology and Genetic Engineering Reviews article by William Freese and David Schubert, "the FDA never sees the methodological details, but rather only limited data and the conclusions the company has drawn from its own research....the FDA does not require the submission of data. And, in fact, companies have failed to comply with FDA requests for data beyond that which they submitted initially. Without test protocols or other important data, the FDA is unable to identify unintentional mistakes, errors in data interpretation, or intentional deception..."

There are really some insane substances companies use, one manufacturer tried to use Hydrogen Peroxide on onions!

Well done FDA...

"Eat less from the box and more from the Earth."

- Unknown

"Every time you eat or drink, you are either feeding disease or fighting it."

- Heather Morgan.

Chapter 7

Would Eating Become an Addiction?

Many people have asked this question - is there such a thing called food addiction or can food be addictive? The simple answer is absolute yes! However, food addiction is growing rapidly and the worst part of this addiction is that no one takes it seriously. Based on the concept of "food" is a not drug or alcohol, it's just food. But the fact is, regardless what the substance is, it is an addiction if you crave for it. Therefore, food can be addictive. Many people are addicted to foods without even knowing or aware of such addiction. And the risks of this addiction are severe based on the growing diseases, cancers and deaths which we're clearly facing these days.

What is an addiction?

Generally, an addiction is referred to any action or behavior someone does which a person has no control over. Usually, there are consequences and these may vary depending on the type of the addiction. According to the medical-dictionary, as well as mainstream psychology, addiction is a persistent, compulsive, dependence on a behavior or substance. The term has been partially replaced by the word dependence for substance abuse. Addiction has been extended, however, to include mood-altering behaviors or activities. Some researchers speak of two types of addictions: substance addictions (i.e. alcoholism, drug abuse, and smoking) and process addictions (e.g. gambling, spending, shopping, eating, and sexual activity etc.) There is a growing recognition that many addicts, such as drugs/polydrug abusers, are addicted to more than one substance or process.

The above definition of addiction, as well as most of the mainstream psychology and behavioral science, categorize the eating addiction only in the "process addictions". However, food addiction can be on the same level as alcohol and drugs category. It's true there are some differences, but they also share lots of similarities.

Food Addiction

The process of how people get addicted to food is complicated, but to sum up the process in simple terms, we need to understand what exactly happens when a person is craving for food, such as the feelings involved as well as the satisfaction afterwards. And also, the reasons of "why" food addiction is more difficult to deal with. When I do weight management counseling sessions with some clients, the lack of acknowledgment and persistence in denying the addiction by the person who is addicted to food is noteworthy. Food addiction shouldn't be underestimated as we cannot underestimate other addictive substances such as alcohol, smoking and drugs.

The consequences of smoking are cancers along with social, economic and other health issues and diseases which may lead to death. Alcohol addictions and abuse will also lead to liver failure along with social and economic consequences and other diseases may lead to death. Drugs' addiction and abuse also goes the same way, social, economic issues and other health problem may lead to death. On the other hand, food addiction goes exactly the same way as the previous three addictions - which may lead to obesity, cancers, diabetes, social issues, economic and other health problems which may also lead to death. But what makes people more prone to food addiction is that people have to eat to survive, unlike smoking, drugs and alcohol. The food addiction is linked to too many physical, biological, social and psychological factors. Many people don't start realizing it until their body shape start to change and their health has declined.

How do people get addicted to food?

Food addiction as stated earlier is a complicated addiction due to the importance of food to us to survive. However, there are few factors involved in food addiction such as physical, biological, social and psychological. This very addiction also involves all our sensors to get "anchored" to foods and eating (an anchor, in this case, is a mental program, and will be explained precisely in the media and psychology chapter). The anchor is being programmed in the mind not only on the taste satisfaction but also on our visual sense, auditory (hearing), kinesthetic (feeling), olfactory (smelling) and gustatory (taste). The addiction starts when a person loses control of what and when to eat, and it's more than just eating mismanagement. To be able to understand the factors that are involved in addiction I'll start first by examining what attracts us to foods, especially junk foods, and how this attraction becomes a habit and the habit leads to addictions.

What attracts us to food and why do we keep eating?

Many people feel guilty after they over eat, especially junk or unhealthy foods. Feeling guilty is a sign of acknowledgement as there is something wrong or that something is not done right. However, when you understand what is in the foods you're eating, the feeling of guilt will turn into a strategy - of how you're going to manage to eat and manage the portion of those addictive food substances.

The three main addictive substances in foods can be simply defined as the three deadly whites - which are sugar, salt and fat. These three are what gets the person addicted and return for more, as will be explained later through the physical, biological, social and psychological factors.

Sugar: The only difference between drugs and sugar is just the legal part. However, there are many studies regarding sugar as an addictive substance and almost all the studies show similar results – which is "yes sugar is addictive". Paul van der Velpen, head of Amsterdam's health department, warns that sugar is a dangerous, addictive drug and sugary foods and soft drinks should be labelled with warning labels similar to those on cigarette packets, except these would be warnings for obesity, diabetes, cancers and other health concerns. The best thing to add to any food product to get people to buy it, again and again, is sugar, and that is the reason of a can of soda drink contains 10 and some brands up to 15 teaspoons of sugar. While the maximum daily amount of an average person according to the American Heart Association (AHA) shouldn't exceed 150 calories per day (37.5 grams or 9 teaspoons) for men and 100 calories per day (25 grams or 6 teaspoons) for women. That amount is for an "average person" not overweight or obese person.

Dr. Leri an Associate Professor of Neuroscience and Applied Cognitive Science at the University of Guelph, Ontario, Canada. Dr. Leri presented a study that caused behavioral reactions in rats linked to the same problems produced by addictive drugs. Dr. Leri stated, "Addiction to unhealthy foods could help explain the global obesity epidemic." Professor Leri also said, "We have evidence in laboratory animals of a shared vulnerability to develop preferences for sweet foods and for cocaine."

David Kessler a former head of the Food and Drug Administration (FDA) believes that sugar is just as addictive as cigarettes and he says that it is "highly pleasurable. It gives you this momentary bliss. When you're eating food that is highly hedonic, it sort of takes over your brain." That is exactly what drugs do, but once again, one is legal and the other is not. This is due to the same old reason as in the ancient book of reasons "follow the money"!

Furthermore, according to Dr. Jennifer Lee, department of Psychology, "Rats addicted to sugar ingest it in a binge-like manner that releases dopamine in the accumbens (the rewarding system in the brain) during and right before consumption, much like heroin use in humans. And also like drug addiction, this sugar bingeing causes changes in the expression and availability of dopamine receptors in the brain: the next "high" will require even more sugar to achieve the same effect."

There are tons of researches and they all state that sugar is as addictive as drugs. It does influence and affects the behavior and it does lead to diabetes, diseases, cancers and death. Sugar is widely available and legal in every food product we buy. According to the Department of Health and Human Services "Today, the average American consumes almost 152 pounds (almost 69 kg) of sugar in one year. This is equal to 3 pounds (or 6 cups) of sugar consumed in one week! Nutritionists suggest that Americans should get only 10% of their calories from sugar. This equals 13.3 teaspoons of sugar per day (based on 2,000 calories per day)." This disaster is still growing. And governments don't seem they are going to put any end to it while the world is run by corporations who run most governments. So, don't wait for a change because it's not going to happen any soon. You must start with yourself and "keep that poison out of the reach of your family and especially children".

More about the effect of sugar can be found in greater detail in the chapter "Sugar the sweet toxin".

Salt: It is yet another drug so addictive as sugar and fat, with too many side effects lead to very serious and deadly health issues. It has found its way to our foods and diet, introduced intentionally to our diet for no other reason but to be addictive, hence, you will return for more.

A team of Duke University Medical Center and Australian scientists has found that salt is a powerfully addictive drug. Research shows how certain genes are structured in a part of the brain that controls the balance of salt, water, energy, reproduction and other rhythms of the hypothalamus (an area of the brain responsible for hormone production). This means salt has a direct link to emotions and behavior just as all other drugs do. The scientists found that the gene patterns activated by stimulating an instinctive behavior, salt appetite, were the same groups of genes regulated by cocaine or opiate (such as heroin) addiction.

According to Wolfgang Liedtke, M.D., Ph.D., a DIBS Investigator and Assistant Professor of Medicine and Neurobiology, "Our findings have profound and far-reaching medical implications, and could lead to a new understanding of addictions and the detrimental consequences when obesity-generating foods are overloaded with sodium."

It is also believed that our craving for salt may be due to evolution, as salt has been known to have the ability to preserve food throughout history as Morris, M.J., Na, E.S., Johnson, A.K. Department of Psychology, the University of Iowa, Iowa City, IA., Physiology & Behavior suggested.

Salt is important in our diet, just as some healthy sugars, but only in small portions; unlike when buying a packet of potato chips where most of the food product is made of salt! Salt is not only found in snacks but in almost every food product you buy. Salt is found in sauces, bread, burgers and even in drinks and energy drinks.

Table Salt (Sodium chloride) is made of 40 percent sodium, an electrolyte that helps to maintain the fluids balance in the body, more specifically in the cells for contracting the muscles and for transmitting nerve impulses. Water tends to move to higher concentrations of sodium, so the more sodium, the more water the body retains. Also, salt helps the digestive system to absorb nutrients. Despite the importance of salt for our bodies, the body needs far less of the amount people consume every day. According to The Centers For Disease Control (CDC) recommends Americans consume no more than 2,300 mg of sodium per day (that about one teaspoon of salt), and those with certain medical conditions (such as high blood pressure) should keep consumption to under 1,500 mg per day. However, the average American consumes about 3,400 mg daily, which can contribute to major heart problems, water retention, dehydration, hypertension, high blood pressure, weakening of bones, increase in weight, hardening of arteries, increase in uric acid, worsening of edema (abnormal accumulation of fluid), bronchial and Lung problems. Also, a low-salt zone leads to stroke, heart attack and death, according to a 2011 study in the Journal of the American Medical Association. Salt (sodium) intake should be kept in moderation. Consult your doctor to check the best amount of the daily intake for you to keep on the safe side. However, the bottom line is, salt is also an addictive substance. It is also added to food to preserve the shelf life of food products; as well as to get you addicted so you keep coming back for more.

Fat: Scientists have confirmed that fatty foods and foods with high-fat content such as ice cream, cheese cake, sausages, bacon, burgers and other fatty foods or with high-calorie foods affect the brain in the same way as cocaine and heroin do.

According to Paul J. Kenny, Ph.D., an associate professor of molecular therapeutics at the Scripps Research Institute, in Jupiter Florida, taking drugs such as cocaine and eating too much junk food, both gradually overload the pleasure centers in the brain and this is exactly what drugs do. And notice how satisfied and relaxed you get when you eat, and how agitated you feel as an addict when you're hungry or craving food. Here's how it works, (as also described in more details in the chapter "why are we getting fat"). We have an area in the brain called Nucleus Accumbens (pleasure and reward system), when an external stimulus, such as a certain foods, drugs and even when you meet a person with a potentially pleasurable sensation, the cerebral cortex signals the ventral tegmental area of the brain to release the chemical dopamine into the amygdala, the prefrontal cortex and the nucleus accumbens. These areas of the brain make up the "reward system". These areas work together to deliver a sense of pleasure and focus the attention of the individual so the individual will learn to repeat the behavior once more. Researchers theorize that this is how behaviors are necessary for survival, reproduction and eating are learned. Cocaine and heroin target and hijack this same reward system. So do food and drugs. Researchers now are considering obesity from the standpoint of addiction. That also explains how the food industry manipulates products by adding so much unnecessary sugar, salt and fat in order to increase consumption by getting the masses addicted to their products. That explains why commercials and advertisements combine food with sex, they are actually targeting that area in the brain Nucleus Accumbens "potential pleasurable sensation". More about the psychology part is explained in the Media chapter.

According to Dr. Gene-Jack Wang, M.D., the chair of the medical department at the U.S. Department of Energy's Brookhaven National Laboratory, in Upton, New York, "We make our food very similar to cocaine now." The fact of getting people addicted to food, especially fat, sugar and salt is no longer a hypothesis or a conspiracy theory - it's a fact, affecting people on a global scale for profit, money and control. According to Kelly Brownell, director of Yale University's Rudd Center for Food Policy & Obesity and a proponent of anti-obesity regulation, "People knew for a long time cigarettes were killing people, but it was only later they learned about nicotine and the intentional manipulation of it." And the same thing is happening with food and all the toxic addictive substances in the food products. Those who are in control work in total secrecy. And those who speak out "the whistle blowers" are usually faced with ridicules by the media and other puppet outlets. This is not a conspiracy, this is fact. These matters about food addictions which are mentioned in this book have been raised in the U.S since the 1990s, but it was believed as a conspiracy orchestrated by those doctors and professors who were first to speak out. They were also ridiculed or silenced exactly as the previous health professionals when they spoke out about the dangers of cigarettes. When people realized it was true - as many deaths were occurring because of tobacco, governments and whoever owns them rushed in to justify it with a couple of researches to say "yes cigarettes cause cancer". As Kelly Brownell said, "People knew for a long time cigarettes were killing people, but it was only later they learned about nicotine and the intentional manipulation of it."

Think about the medical care costs of obesity, this is staggering. ONLY in the United States, in 2008 these costs totaled around $147 billion USD, according to National Library of Medicine National Institutes of Health, Annual medical spending attributable to obesity, Health Affairs in 2009. That was in 2009 when the population count was less than today. Also, obesity is clearly growing on the daily bases rather than declining. $147 billion is a very profitable business to those corporations and those who support them. Yet, you, I and our children and families are paying the bigger bill. The price we pay is priceless, it's our health and wellbeing.

We eat to live not live to eat

It is one of the best proverbs to be said when it comes to food and eating. It means we should eat only to survive and not to allow eating to become a habit. With the quality of foods we have today, eating will certainly become a very bad habit and followed by worse consequences. The main point balances, and to apply this concept to eating is very simple - eat only when you are hungry and only when you need to eat, but it's not normal to be hungry all the time, and if you feel that you're hungry more than the usual, that could be a sign either psychological (addiction) or physically (health) as a problem.

There is a technique that I often tell people about - before you eat just take a minute to think, why am I eating? Am I really hungry? How much do I really need to eat to be safe and to keep my body running? Just a few questions you could ask yourself to raise your awareness and to keep your mind focused on the amount of food and the types of foods you're eating. And also to keep yourself within the boundaries of a healthy meal. The mind is so powerful when you acknowledge its powers. "Mens sana in corpore sano"- a healthy mind in a healthy body.

More about suggestions will be in the "the suggestions" chapter.

"My drug of choice is food. I use food for the same reasons an addict uses drugs: to comfort, to soothe, to ease stress."

– Oprah Winfrey

"Being addicted to food brings suffering, declining health and total lack of self-esteem."

– Deepak Chopra

Chapter 8
Sugar the Sweet Toxins

Nowadays, there are two types of sweet poisons which have been wedged into our diets as well as into almost every product we consume – sugar and high fructose corn syrup HFCS. Those two sweet poisons are causing enormous metabolic issues didn't exist before when we used to consume complex carbohydrates.

A recent analysis associated with the International Diabetes Federation Database, indicated while experimental and observational studies suggest that sugar intake is associated with developing type 2 diabetes. The analysis shows the only thing associated with the increase is sugar. That proves the main point, which is a calorie is not a calorie as it's believed in general, because according to Dr. Lustig sugar is 40 - 50 times more potent than total calories, and that explains the global diabetes rate.

Also, Dr. Lustig indicated, one of the major problems which also play a major role in moving the world toward obesity and other diseases is when we combine fat and carbohydrates together in the same food. If you notice, almost all the foods and food products we consume these days contain a combination of fat and carbohydrates together. Sugar has its unique composition, and the sugar that is available now is the only food on the planet which contains fat and carbohydrates. If you look at fatty foods in nature such as avocado, olive, coconut and similar foods, they contain fat but not carbohydrates. There are no eatable plants on this planet that have fat and carbohydrates combined in the same plant (fruit and vegetable). It's always one or the other.

Some people wonder if there's fat in sugar! Well, if you do a simple research on sugar, you'll find that sugar is made up of two molecules, the first one is called Glucose and the second one is Fructose.

Dr. Lusting further explains about glucose and fructose, **Glucose** is not that sweet, interesting and appealing to humans to crave it or get addicted to it. Glucose is metabolized by all the organs in the body. Every single organism on the face of the earth can digest, absorb and metabolize glucose because it's the energy of life, and if you don't have glucose in your diet, your body will make it because all your cells need it to function. And also, 80% of the glucose you take in - is metabolized by all the organs in your body and only 20% of it goes to the liver.

On the other hand, **Fructose** is very sweet, very interesting to us, we crave it and look for it in foods and we are very likely to get addicted to it. Fructose can only be metabolized by the liver because only the liver has the transporting mechanisms for fructose - which means all the fructose goes only to the liver. In other words, you're overloading the liver with fructose. And here is the process - the fructose goes straight to the mitochondria, it is turned into fat, and with a little bit of glucose, it goes to glycogen until it's complete and it goes to fat as well. Then the result will be mitochondria meltdown or disease; when you have mitochondria disease you get very sick. Therefore, fructose is a chronic hepato-toxin (liver toxin) just like alcohol. In fact, fructose is more like alcohol than anything else! Alcohol is metabolized to fat, and in the same way as fructose, driving more liver fat that can export more liver insulin resistance. This process pushes the pancreas to make more insulin, leading to energy deposition into fat cells and essentially leading to weight-gain. The extra insulin leads to high blood pressure, causing heart disease, activating cell division, (which leads to cancer), changes in the brain leads to dementia and when your pancreas can't make enough of this insulin; it runs out and leads to diabetes as well. Also, what's more, interesting is; if you look at the diseases of alcohol, sugar, and obesity they are all the same! However, fructose and alcohol are both nutrients and can supply us with energy, because they are natural and if you're starving or glycogen depleted in some cases, such as running a marathon - fructose and alcohol can be used to rebuild your energy stores, and in that case, they are not toxins. If you're not glycogen depleted or if you are not running a marathon, then what your liver cells will do with both fructose and alcohol - is to turn them into liver fat and then it's a dangerous toxin.

Some people believe there's no harm or risks in adding sugar to foods, but the fact is when you add sugar to packaged and processed foods, you'll make the problem worse, and that is what is killing us today – besides the toxic environment that we have created.

We have shaped the world in the last few decades into this extremely oversized world. If you think about what the excessive use of bad sugar have resulted in the last few decades and think about another few decades from now with whatever diseases we already have, then imagine what the result would be!

Corn syrup sweeteners, soft drinks and beverages

Sadly, people nowadays drink soft drinks more than they drink water. Soft drinks have become a part of almost every meal. Every food outlet, restaurant, junk food restaurant etc. have a package deal that comes with soft drink. People don't know what lurks behind every sip of that drink, what it is made of, and the subsequent risks in combining such ingredients.

I'll start first with the sugar in the soft drinks; whether it's a juice, flavored soda, cola, energy drink, even the-so-claimed vitamins in water drinks.

Any beverage you buy has a similar amount of sugar, regardless of its brand and flavor. Let's take for example 12 oz. (355 ml) can of cola or soda drink. It contains around 40g of sugar - which is approximately 10 teaspoons of sugar. The bottle of 20 oz (590 ml) soda drink contains between 65 - 77g of sugar, depends on the brand! You can use this simple universal measurement of 4 grams = 1 teaspoons.

Another example is when you go to a fast food restaurant and order a meal - comes with a large cola or other flavored drink. You will get around 55g (around 14 teaspoons) for the medium and an enormous 76 grams (19 teaspoons) for the large drink. That's only in the drink. The amount of sugar in the meal such as bread, sauce, chips, fries, dessert, etc. is not included, so you have to add the extra amount of sugars with the rest of that meal.

Also, a cinema serving soft drink contains approximately 23 teaspoons of sugar, while the large one contains 44 teaspoons of sugar (not 44 grams!!! It's 44 TEASPOONS of sugar) each to be consumed within approximately 90 min or less. This is an insane amount of sugar in only ONE drink to watch a movie. If you add the amount of sugar in the popcorn and other confectioneries such as chocolate etc. along with the 44 teaspoons (176 grams), you'll end up with a disaster. Let's do a simple calculation; 176 grams of sugar in the large drink + 120 grams in large popcorn + 50 grams in any kind of confectioneries = around 346 grams of sugar! That's almost a 100 grams over a quarter of a kilo (0.760 pound) = (86.5 teaspoons of sugar) – while the recommended daily intake of sugar is maximum 37.5 grams (9 teaspoons) for men and 25 grams (6 teaspoons) for women, per day according to the American Heart Association (AHA).

Moreover, since soft drinks are the largest source of calories in the Western World's diet, on November 1984, the largest soft drink companies replaced their sugar with corn syrup, and since then the high fructose corn syrup found its new host to – the people's bloodstream. The main reason for the big companies to switch from natural sugar to high fructose corn syrup sweetener was because "it's cheaper". The saving from that switch has made enormous profits for those companies. The bottles and cups started to get larger, and the consumption of the individual got larger as well - from 350 cans a year to almost 600 cans a year according to statistics.

The dangers of High Fructose Corn Syrup (HFCS) and Artificial Sweeteners

High Fructose Corn Syrup HFCS is a cheap sweetener that has undergone enzymatic processing to convert some of its glucose into fructose to produce a desired sweetness. Due to its low price compared to sugar, it is also the predominant sweetener used in processed foods, bread, cereals, yoghurt, baked food, canned food, lunch meat, dairy products and many other processed and packaged foods and beverages. HFCS have been used in our foods since the 1980s.

HFCS is among other sweeteners have primarily replaced sucrose (table sugar) in the food industry. It was a great idea in the United States to replace the sucrose with HFCS due to the production of corn in the 1970s. This was during Nixon's presidential time, which was the reasons for this to be included in governmental production quotas of domestic sugar, subsidies of U.S. corn, and an import tariff on foreign sugar. All of which combine to raise the price of sucrose to levels above those of the rest of the world, and making HFCS the cheapest option for many sweetener applications.

Furthermore, now HFCS exists in almost every food product and has replaced sucrose - which is also unhealthy - and that left us with no other choice but to go from bad to worse. It's not a matter of debate anymore regarding the risks, or the lack of nutritional benefits for humans in consuming HFCS and other sweeteners as the negative results and the consequences of those sweeteners are already have been proven.

According to the American Society for Clinical Nutrition, in the United States, HFCS has primarily been used to substitute for sucrose as a caloric sweetener, rather than to be used in addition to sucrose. Sucrose use has declined from 80% of total caloric sweetener availability in 1970 to 40% of caloric sweetener availability in 1997. This reduction in sucrose consumption was simply because of the switch to HFCS - which has increased from nearly 0% in 1970 to 40% of total caloric sweeteners in 1997. The availability of HFCS in the US food supply did not change from 1997 [60.4 pounds (27.4 kg) per capita annually]. The same journal also states "there is no evidence that the ratio of fructose and glucose consumed from sugars has changed over the past four decades as a result of HFCS replacing sucrose in many applications." That means the result is the same in the usage of HFCS till today, but obviously, obesity, diabetes and other diseases have dramatically increased.

Thanks to the media for running their skillful deceptions and campaigns through the Corn Refiners Accusation, and others who are benefiting by telling the world that the harm of HFCS is nothing but a myth or a conspiracy. This is while using smart media spins denying the studies and journals of medical and nutritional experts as it is "nothing but some researches personal opinion". Essentially, trying to convince the masses about the safety to consume HFCS as it is a "natural" sweetener extracted from natural corn - as sucrose is extracted from sugar canes and it's totally safe for humans' consumption if it is used in moderation. However, if this is their argument, then why the corn industry is spending millions of dollars on their misinformation and deception campaigns to convince the people and health professionals about the safety of their products?

The science behind the dangers of HFCS and sugar

If we're going to compare which of the two is more natural than the other - sugar canes or HFCS, simply, both are far from being natural based in their biochemistry process and the way they are produced.

Cane-sugar: White crystal sugar and sugar cubes are not picked from trees and definitely brown sugar doesn't come from honey. Sugar must pass a chemical process to make the sugar white, brown raw or cubes. According to Pigman and Horton, The Carbohydrates: Chemistry and Biochemistry, sugar usually refers to all carbohydrates of the general formula $Cn(H2O)n$. Sucrose is a disaccharide, or double sugar, composed of one molecule of glucose linked to one molecule of fructose. Because one molecule of water ($H2O$) is lost in the condensation reaction linking glucose to fructose, sucrose is represented by the formula $C12\ H22\ O11$ (with a chemical formula of $C12\ H22\ O11$) and it can be broken down into a molecule of glucose ($C6H12O6$) plus a molecule of fructose (also $C6H12O6$, an isomer of glucose), in a weakly acidic environment by a process called inversion. Sucrose is broken down during digestion into a mixture of 50% fructose and 50% glucose through hydrolysis by the enzyme sucrose (enzymes). People with Sucrose deficiency cannot digest (break down) sucrose and thus exhibit sucrose intolerance. There is nothing natural about the sucrose (table sugar) you're consuming, it is a substance with a biochemical process.

High Fructose Corn Syrup HFCS: According to White JS., HFCS starts with corn; the corn will be milled to produce starch-corn starch. The process of making corn syrup from starch, the cornstarch is mixed with water ($H2O$) and then an enzyme will be added, produced by a bacterium that breaks the starch down into shorter chains of glucose. Then another enzyme, produced by a fungus breaks down the short chains into glucose molecules. At that point, regular corn syrup is made. Moreover, when converting the corn syrup into high fructose corn syrup, some of its glucose molecules will be turned into fructose molecules by exposing the syrup to yet another enzyme, again produced by bacteria. This enzyme converts the glucose to a mixture of about 42 percent fructose and 53 percent glucose, with some other sugars as well. This syrup, called HFCS 42, is as sweet as sucrose (table sugar) and it is used in foods, pastry and bakery products. HFCS 55, which contains approximately 55 percent fructose and 42 percent glucose, is sweeter than sucrose and sugar made from sugar canes. HFCS is also cheaper than sugar, because of the government farm bill corn subsidies. This allowed the average soda size to dramatically increase from 8 ounces (226.7 ml) to 20 ounces (570 ml) with a small financial cost to the manufacturers.

As I already explained in the previous chapter, fructose goes straight to the liver and triggers lipogenesis which is the production of fats like triglycerides and cholesterol. It causes a condition called "fatty liver" which affects 10-24% of the general population, according to U.S national Library of Medicine, National Institute of Health.

Also, the constant absorption of glucose triggers a major shot of insulin in the body's main fat storage hormone. Both of these structures of HFCS lead to increased metabolic imbalance which increases the appetite, weight gain, diabetes, heart disease, cancer, dementia, and many more diseases.

According to a test done by the Institute for Agriculture and Trade Policy and other researchers, including an FDA researcher - they have found HFCS often contains toxic levels of mercury, because of color-alkali products used in the manufacturing process. In case you don't know, mercury is toxic and it damages the nervous system. It is one of the primary risks for pregnant women and their fetuses. That's the main reasons pregnant mothers and infants are encouraged to avoid seafood.

Mercury also causes vision problems, as well as impairment of speech, walking and muscle weakness and other issues. Some people have insomnia, headaches, emotional issues and skin problems due to mercury poisoning. And it's also been linked to autism, ADD and AD. Furthermore, the contamination of corn syrup with mercury as the research shows, four of the big plants that make corn syrup use mercury-cell technology in the production of caustic soda, an ingredient used in the corn conversion process. It's a very technical process, but the bottom line is; mercury is being found in food products, and mercury can cause severe brain imbalances. The results also found that a strange chemical appeared during the tests are not glucose or fructose. This certainly calls into question the purity of this processed form of this sugar. The exact nature, effects, and toxicity of these odd compounds have not been fully explained, but shouldn't we be protected from the presence of untested chemical compounds in our food supply, especially since HFCS is infested in almost all of our food supply?

The risks of HFCS and sugar, in general, are countless. HFCS contributes to various other health issues beside obesity, such as; insulin resistance, elevated blood pressure, elevated triglycerides and elevated LDL, depletion of vitamins and minerals, cardiovascular disease, liver disease, cancer, arthritis, and even gout. There are numerous of studies have proven that HFCS is not safe for the consumption of humans - and yet, the FDA isn't going to do anything about it. As a matter of fact, the FDA considers HFCS as GRAS (Generally Regarded As Safe) regardless of all the existed data and studies which detected unsafe mercury levels in HFCS, the crystalline fructose, the super-potent form of fructose etc. The food and beverage industry is using HFCS despite the presence of arsenic, lead, chloride and heavy metals. Also, in addition to the fact that nearly all the corn used to make the HFCS is made from genetically modified corn, which already comes with its own set of risks.

What else does science say about the health impact of fructose?

According to GreenMedInfo.com as well as countless other researches and scientific studies, they have linked fructose to almost 30 different specific diseases and health problems including:

Raises your blood pressure and causes nocturnal hypertension	Insulin resistance / Type 2 Diabetes	Non-alcoholic fatty liver disease (NAFLD)
Raises your uric acid levels which can result in gout and/or metabolic syndrome	Accelerates the progression of chronic kidney disease	Intracranial atherosclerosis (narrowing and hardening of the arteries in your skull)
Exacerbates cardiac abnormalities if you're deficient in copper	Have a genotoxic effect on the colon	Promotes metastasis in breast cancer patients

Causes tubulointerstitial injury (injury to the tubules and interstitial tissue of your kidney)	Promotes obesity and related health problems and diseases	Promotes pancreatic cancer growth and feeds cancer cells in general
Causes your brain neurons to stagnate		

Now you know about sugar cane sucrose and HFCS and you know about their risks on your health and weight. Therefore, you might be planning to switch your normal beverage to zero sugar or diet drink and your food to diet or light. However, there is another enemy maybe worse than all, lurking in the dark behind those words such as zero sugar, sugar-free, light and diet etc. This enemy, by all means, is a ruthless killer, made in labs to confuse the minds of people and deceive their taste buds. This enemy is called "Aspartame".

Aspartame:

Aspartame is the technical name for the brand names NutraSweet®, Equal, Spoonful, and Equal-Measure. The NutraSweet® company profile is that aspartame was discovered by accident in 1965 when James Schlatter, a chemist of G.D. Searle Company who was testing an anti-ulcer drug. Searle was bought by "Monsanto" in 1985 and then on May 25th, 2000 - J.W. Childs Equity Partners II L.P. purchased the NutraSweet® Company from Monsanto, a wholly owned subsidiary of Pharmacia Corporation.

According to the U.S. National Library of Medicine/ the National Institutes of Health (NIH), Aspartame is 220 times sweeter than sugar. It's not a mystery that people like sugar, it's simply because they have become addicted to it. Each person consumes about 152 pounds (almost 69 kg) of sugars per year on average, according to the Department of Health and Human Services. Most of that sugar is added sugar, and for most people, it comes from soda and other sugary beverages. In 1981 Aspartame was approved for dry goods, and two years later in 1983 became approved for carbonated beverages. It was originally approved for dry goods on July 26, 1974, but objections filed by a neuroscience researcher Dr. John W. Olney and consumer attorney James Turner in August 1974, as well as investigations of G.D. Searle's research practices, caused the U.S. Food and Drug Administration (FDA) to put approval of Aspartame on hold on December 5, 1974.

In 1985 Monsanto purchased G.D. Searle, the chemical company that held the patent to aspartame, the active ingredient in NutraSweet®. Certainly, Monsanto knew its past before they purchased it, especially the 1980 confirmation of the three independent scientists with FDA Board of Inquiry, which confirmed that "Aspartame might induce brain tumors." The FDA had actually banned aspartame based on this finding, research on areas such as neurological functions, brain tumors, seizures, headaches, and adverse effects on children and pregnant women, and here are the Grist reports:

"In a 1996 survey, Ralph G. Walton ... looked at 166 peer-reviewed studies on aspartame undertaken between 1980 and 1985. He found that all 74 of the studies funded by the industry found no adverse effects from aspartame, while 84 of the 92 independently funded articles did find bad effects."

What is Aspartame and how did it get FDA safe approval?

Aspartame is the ingredient found in NutraSweet®. It is also found in Equal, Spoonful, Equal-Measure, AminoSweet, Benevia, NutraTaste, Canderel, and many popular "diet" sodas. This chemical is currently on the ingredient list of nearly 6,000 products worldwide. But since it was approved for use as a food additive in 1981, it has been dogged by complaints about its safety.

According to Dr. John Olney, Aspartame was never proven safe for human consumption before it gained FDA approval as a food additive. Dr. Olney believes Aspartame should not be on the market today "because it hasn't been demonstrated to be safe." Also in agreement with Dr. Olney, when the FDA was presented with Dr. Olney's research, they assigned an outside public board of inquiry the task of deciding if aspartame should be allowed for human consumption. In 1980, the doctors on that board unanimously ruled that aspartame should not go on the market. An internal FDA panel concluded the same thing in 1980.

According to the FDA Chairman at that time, Dr. Gere Goyan, his next recommendation was to another FDA committee to study Aspartame. He appointed individuals who had never done or were a part of any former studies of aspartame. Dr. Gere Goyan never saw the results of that 1980 FDA internal study because he was forced to step down as FDA Chairman the day Ronald Reagan took office on January 21, 1981, and his replacement was Dr. Arthur Hill Hayes.

Dr. Hayes had no previous history of dealing with the science of food additives and he was apparently hand-picked to head the FDA by a prominent member of Ronald Reagan's political transition team who was Donald Rumsfeld. Yes, it is the same Donald Rumsfeld who led the United States into the multi trillion-dollar wars in Iraq and Afghanistan, as Secretary of Defense during the Bush administration. But Rumsfeld in 1981 had a different title. He was the CEO of the G.D Searle Company, the company that owned the patent on aspartame.

Moreover, one of Dr. Arthur Hill Hayes first acts as FDA Chairman was granting Aspartame approval for use in dry goods. Also maybe incidentally, one of Hayes' last acts in office as FDA Chairman was to approve aspartame for use in beverages.

Now I wonder, was aspartame approved because studies showed it was safe for human consumption? Or was it approved - thanks to the political influence of Donald Rumsfeld and others?

According to former senator Howard Metzenbaum, who reviewed the FDA's approval process of aspartame in the Senate in 1987, "I think there were a lot of politics involved in its being approved." Research scientist Dr. Olney is even blunter, "the issue Aspartame is really not an issue of science; it's an issue of politics."

The dangers and side effects of Aspartame

The Department of Health and Human Services on April 20, 1995, filed complaints and submitted to the FDA symptoms attributed to Aspartame showing over 92 different health side effects associated with Aspartame consumption.

According to Dr. Lendon Smith, M.D. there is an enormous population suffering from side effects associated with aspartame, yet have no idea why drugs, supplements and herbs don't provide relief from their symptoms. Then, there are users who don't 'appear' to suffer immediate reactions at all. Even these individuals are susceptible to the long-term damage caused by excitatory amino acids, phenylalanine, methanol, and DKP.

Adverse reactions and side effects of aspartame include:

Headaches/ migraines	Dizziness	Seizures	Nausea	Numbness
Muscle spasms	Weight gain	Rashes	Depression	Fatigue
Irritability	Tachycardia	Insomnia	Vision problems	Hearing loss
Heart palpitations	Breathing difficulties	Anxiety attacks	Slurred speech	Loss of taste
Tinnitus	Vertigo	Memory loss	Joint pain	

According to researchers and physicians studying the adverse effects of Aspartame, the following chronic illnesses can be triggered or worsened by ingesting aspartame:

Brain tumors	Multiple sclerosis	Epilepsy	Chronic fatigue syndrome	Parkinson's disease
Alzheimer's	Mental	Lymphoma	Birth	Fibromyalgia

	retardation		defects	
Diabetes				

What's the alternative and solution?

Ideally, it's recommended that you avoid as much sugar as you possibly can, especially if you are overweight or have diabetes, high cholesterol, or high blood pressure. I also understand and know that we don't live in a perfect world, and following a strict food diet program is not always practical or even possible. Once again, I'm not an ND or an MD. You can always check with your doctor/physician regarding what works better for you. However, through the researches that I've done I have found, if you want to use a sweetener occasionally, this is what is recommended:

- Use the herb Stevia.
- Use organic cane sugar in moderation.
- Use organic raw honey in moderation.
- Avoid all artificial sweeteners.
- Avoid Agave syrup since it is a highly processed sap that is almost in all fructose. Your blood sugar will spike just as it would if you were consuming regular sugar or HFCS. Agave's meteoric rise in popularity is due to a great marketing campaign, but any health benefits present in the original agave plant are processed out.
- Avoid the so-called energy drinks and sports drinks because they are loaded with sugar, sodium, and chemical additives. Rehydrating with pure, fresh water is a better choice.

You can always research what works for you, and I highly recommend you to ask your doctor what is best for you and your condition especially if you already have heart problems, low/high blood pressure problems, cholesterol, diabetes or any other medical condition. And I do believe there are still some good and honest medical doctors who don't promote products in their practices based on some personal gains offered to them at the conferences they attend.

Sadly, some doctors have become a marketing media tool for the corporations and their products whether intentionally, or just because they've been told "it's a good product" by the medical boards. Often these conferences have political ties attached to them and are run by the same corporations. However, I still believe in a number of honest doctors and fellow professionals who serve people and are saving lives at their practices, not running a business or an enterprise. These professionals are honest and believe in what they do to assist people, as they have sworn an oath to perform their duties honestly and sincerely.

"Homicide is 0.8% of deaths. Diet-related disease is over 60%. But no one fucking talks about it."

- Jamie Oliver

"I give you bitter pills, in a sugar coating. The pills are harmless - the poison's in the sugar."

- James St. James

Chapter 9
Hungry or Angry = Hangry

You're hungry, starting to feel your energy dropping, you get grumpy and angry even at the silliest things. You have a shorter temper and ready to snap angrily at anything or anyone. Or maybe someone has snapped angrily at you when they were hungry. If so, you've experienced "hangry". Hangry is (an amalgamation of hungry and angry) – the phenomenon by which some people get angry, grumpy and short-tempered when their gustatorial temptations are ready for nourishment and the stomach is overdue for a feed.

According to researchers, when people are hungry, they are more likely to be angry or aggressive because of serotonin. Serotonin is a hormone that regulates every type of behavior, such as appetitive, emotional, motor, cognitive and autonomic. Serotonin levels will fluctuate when people are under stress or even hungry.

According to researchers, the University of Cambridge, Biological Psychiatry journal, states "Fluctuations of serotonin levels in the brain, which often occur when someone hasn't eaten or is stressed, affects brain regions that enable people to regulate anger, new research from the University of Cambridge has shown. Although reduced serotonin levels have previously been implicated in aggression, this is the first study which has shown how this chemical helps regulate behavior in the brain as well as why some individuals may be more prone to aggression."

Also, according to co-first author, Molly Crockett, who worked on the research as a Ph.D. student at Cambridge's Behavioral and Clinical Neuroscience Institute, "We've known for decades that serotonin plays a key role in aggression, but it's only very recently that we've had the technology to look into the brain and examine just how serotonin helps us regulate our emotional impulses. By combining a long tradition in behavioral research with new technology, we were finally able to uncover a mechanism for how serotonin might influence aggression."

A study was performed regarding the effects of serotonin levels. Researchers controlled the diet of healthy volunteers to control and manipulate their serotonin levels. The participants' brains were scanned using functional magnetic resonance imaging (fMRI) as they viewed faces with different expressions such as angry, sad and neutral faces to determine how various parts of their brains reacted and communicated with each other.

The study showed low levels of serotonin made communications between certain parts of the brain weaker than normal. Researchers concluded that when this happens it may be harder for the brain to control emotional responses to anger.

There was also a personality test for the volunteers to assess if they had a natural tendency towards aggression or not. Researchers found those that were easily agitated had even weaker communication between certain areas of their brain when serotonin levels were low.

It was suggested that the result could be applied to a range of psychiatric disorders in which violence is a common problem, such as intermittent explosive disorder, which is characterized by extreme and uncontrollable outbursts of violence.

What is Serotonin?

According to Bristol University in England, Serotonin is a neurotransmitter. Neurotransmitters are chemical substances which transmit nerve impulses across synapses, and synapses are the spaces in between nerve cells. Nerve cells are also known as neurons.

Moreover, serotonin is a chemical messenger that's believed to act as a mood stabilizer and influence our behaviors and mood. It is also known as the happiness hormone because it contributes to the feelings of well-being. Serotonin is involved in our appetite, sleep, memory, learning, temperature, mood, behavior, muscle contraction, depression, cardiovascular function, endocrine regulation, regulates ageing, bone metabolism and wound healing (serotonin is a growth factor for some types of cells).

Another interesting thing about serotonin is - according to researchers at the Maryland University Medical Center, serotonin appears to play a role in causing migraines or headache when someone is hungry. Similarly, other researches also relate low serotonin to feeling cold when hungry. Therefore, we tend to eat more in winter, and consequently, we add on the extra pounds during winter simply because food makes us warm.

On a similar note, winter – cold – hungry – leading to adding some extra pounds in winter. As a result, notice the diet and weight loss commercials usually start buzzing around the beginning of summer. The use of such media spin in that particular time isn't only because people want to look good in summer, but also because of the illusion that such diet programs or products may work. Therefore, there's no magic if you lose few extra pounds in summer by following a commercialized diet program or product, because you'll naturally lose weight in summer with or without a weight loss scam since you don't eat as much in summer.

The relation between Serotonin and depression

Scientists believe that serotonin is involved in making people with depression feel sad, but they still don't know exactly how.

However, the link between serotonin and depression is not fully understood yet, and it is still controversial at this point. Many researchers believe low levels of serotonin cause depression while some other researchers believe other chemical imbalances or brain abnormalities cause depression and this leads to low serotonin levels. Yet another group of researchers believe the truth is somewhere in between those two theories. Despite the argument between the theories, researchers do agree that low serotonin is somehow connected to such psychological problems as depression, anxiety, seasonal affective disorder, and obsessive-compulsive disorder. They further agree - increasing serotonin levels in the body can help relieve the symptoms of these conditions.

There are many researchers who believe, an imbalance in serotonin levels may influence the mood in a way that leads to depression. Possible problems include low brain cell production of serotonin, a lack of receptor sites to enable receiving the serotonin that is made, the inability of serotonin to reach the receptor sites, or a shortage in tryptophan (the chemical where serotonin is made). If any of these biochemical glitches occur, researchers believe it can lead to depression, as well as obsessive-compulsive disorder OCD, anxiety, panic, and even anger.

However, researchers don't know whether the dip in serotonin causes the depression, or the depression causes serotonin levels to drop. Although it is widely believed that serotonin deficiency plays a role in depression, there is no way to measure its levels in the living brain. The antidepressant medications that work on serotonin levels SSRIs (selective serotonin reuptake inhibitors) and SNRIs (serotonin and norepinephrine reuptake inhibitors) are believed to reduce symptoms of depression, but exactly how they work is not yet fully understood.

Note

Now we know that low levels of serotonin and its effect on our behavior and moods. Also, the mood swing when we're hungry and the relations between serotonin and eating when we're sad, feeling lonely, moody, cold, board, feeling down, depressed etc. However, some people may ask - why do we also eat when we are happy as in social gatherings, or when being entertained such as when watching TV or in cinema etc. This can be explained as a pattern or an "Anchor", which will be further explained in greater depth when we get to the psychological factors chapter.

(hang-gree) hangry:

adj. A state of anger caused by a lack of food; hunger causing a negative change in an emotional state.

"Hunger and a lack of blood-corpuscles take all the manhood from a man."

- H.G. Wells

Chapter 10

Depressed Animals = Depressed Humans

A chapter disclaimer:

This chapter contains some sensitive materials about animal cruelty, diets, religious and political stand points as well as other organizations and establishments. If you are sensitive to such materials, then, considering skipping this chapter may be a good choice for you.

Furthermore, I'm NOT an advocate for vegetarianism, veganism, specific lifestyle, diet, religions or movements - nor do I work for any of them or against them. I believe in freedom and freedom of choice as long as there's no harm on oneself, others and other earthlings. I'm also not an advocate nor do I support choices or actions which promote violently and cause disharmony amongst the human family.

I believe, every individual is responsible for the choices they make and I believe there is still a slight chance of hope.

In early 1800s Jean Anthelme Brillat-Savarin wrote, "Dis-Moi ce que tu manges, je te dirai ce que tu es." *Translated from French* - "Tell me what you eat, and I will tell you what you are."

As a result, it is a scientifically proven fact that our food choices affect our health, spirituality, psychology and physiology. The old saying, we are what we eat, is essentially true. Every cell in our body was created from the food we eat, the water we drink and the air we breathe. In addition to nourishing our bodies, food also affects the quality of our lives, our appearance, weight, thinking, moods, energy, the ageing process and our overall health and well-being. Furthermore, since animals share similar biology and behavior as we do, they also become what they eat. Hence, the food and treatment we give to animals and since we consume them and their products – this have a direct effect on our own bodies, behavior and well-being in general.

Think of it this way, consuming an animal or an animal product came from an animal that was deprived in terms of proper nutrients, proper treatment, sick, beaten and depressed will essentially have negative effects on whoever consumes it. Moreover, since animals also become the products of their environments, every cell in their body is also created from the food they eat, the water they drink and the air they breathe. On a similar note, to nourishing their bodies, food and treatments also affect the quality of their well-being which well be passed to the consumer and also will affect the consumer on many different levels! In other words, if you're consuming a sick animal (psychologically/physically), you'll also be affected and get sick. And the same thing goes when consuming a depressed animal.

Animals and emotions

Sadly, some scientists and people, in general, believe that cognitive thinking and emotions are exclusive only to humans. I've also came across some scientific publications claim that only humans can speak, laugh, cry, think, suffer from mental disorders such as depression and schizophrenia, choose partners and fall in love. Well, that is utterly nonsense! Animals do communicate and simply no need to elaborate on that. Animals do laugh as scientifically proven by many researchers including the research of Patricia Simonet whose work on dog laughter has been well accepted in the scientific community.

Crying, in the sense of weeping producing emotional tears, yes, humans maybe the only species to produce emotional tears but that's because humans crying has a social or performative nature. Humans are species of drama and art evolved to cry in such a way as a performance of expression. However, all mammals make distress calls, and as Professor Ad Vingerhoets from Tilburg University explains "like when an offspring is separated from its mother, but only humans cry." We can't compare human's crying to animals, simply because the method of crying is not the point but the distress call is!

Thinking, the claim that animals can't think is utterly ludicrous. In fact, animals are well able to think and to behave rationally. Otherwise, hunting and hiding wouldn't have anything to do with strategies and would be solely instincts. Lions can measure the distance and the speed of the prey before attacking. Orang-a-tang apes can use a spear for fishing. Crows have learned to drop nuts from wires onto pedestrian crosswalks. They let the cars crush the nuts, then wait for the green pedestrians crossing light to fly down and retrieve the nuts before the light changes. There are countless of other animal behavior exhibiting an extra-ordinary complex way of thinking.

Suffering, from mental disorders such as depression and schizophrenia, researchers such as physician Hope Ferdowsian and psychologist Gay Bradshaw, have shown that captive animals do indeed suffer a wide range of psychological disorders including post-traumatic stress disorder PTSD. Countless animals are being used and abused in a wide range of human venues. And indeed, researchers continue to use animal models of depression and other psychological conditions to try to learn more about similar disorders in humans. More about animal suffering are detailed in this chapter.

Partnership and falling in love, I'm not sure where to begin here because there are so many examples of animals falling in love and remaining in love for long periods of time. Individuals of many different species form long-term and extremely close social bonds characterized by clear affection and attachment that we call love in human animals.

They clearly miss one another when they are separated and suffer from the absence of individuals with whom they're closely bonded. We see love among mated pairs and also between parents and their children and among members of a group. Of course, one can pitch a definition of love so high so as to exclude many humans but accepted definitions of the word "love" clearly apply to other animals.

Animal's depression and stress lead them to suicide

As stated earlier that animals also have feelings, they do get depressed and even do commit suicide in some cases of depression.

There are lots of debate regarding animal's suicide. On the contrary, there is also some evidence are worth to study. For example, lovebirds - when one of the partners dies before the other mate, the remaining bird starves itself to death, and prior to its certain death, the bird refuses to sing or make any noise. And there are endless other similar examples.

Once again, this topic is "scientifically" controversial based on the hypothesis of, "if animals have rational instinct" or "if animals deliberately end their lives based on a decision, not an instinct". However, there are many cases indicate that some animals deliberately end their lives for reasons as humans do. There are numerous stories regarding animals and pets ending their lives clearly based on stressful situations, as well as going through depression, and also in some cases could be part of their lifecycle. For example, a dog will starve itself to death when its owner dies, a gold fish repeatedly tries to jump out the fish tank (aquarium) to die after its mate has died, and the cases of mass animal suicides. Another example, dolphins and whales committing suicide when they repeatedly beach themselves offshore to die, even after multiple times of human rescuing them. That could be just lemmings, but could also be based on some deliberate and intelligent decision.

Here is the famous story of Kathy the dolphin. Kathy was a depressed dolphin and committed suicide by an intentional asphyxiation. Richard O'Barry a dolphin trainer in the 1960s on the television show "Flipper" says "She (Kathy the dolphin) was really depressed. You have to understand dolphins and whales are not [involuntary] air breathers as we are. Every breath they take is a conscious effort. They can end their lives whenever." Also, "She [Kathy] swam into my arms and looked me right in the eye, took a breath and didn't take another one. I let her go and she sank straight down on her belly to the bottom of the tank." That experience transformed Richard O'Barry, the dolphin trainer, into an animal rights activist and made him a celebrity after his role in "The Cove," an Oscar-winning documentary. He also stated "the [animal entertainment] industry doesn't want people to think dolphins are capable of suicide, but these are self-aware creatures with a brain larger than a human brain. If life becomes so unbearable, they just don't take the next breath. It's suicide."

Animal suicide may seem absurd to some people, however, if we go back during the Greek philosophy era and more specifically Aristotle's time we can see other examples. Aristotle told a story about a stallion that jumped into an abyss after realizing it was deceived into mating with its own mother, and the topic was discussed by early Christian theologians and Victorian academics. Duncan Wilson, a medical historian at the University of Manchester and co-author of a study in the March issue of the British journal Endeavour on the history of self-destructive animals, stated, "The questioning of animal suicide is essentially people looking at what it means to be human".

Moreover, in Britain during the 19th century, after Charles Darwin established the theory of evolution, humane societies formed, vegetarianism and pets became popular, and reports of animal suicide started to reappear again. The usual suspect this time was a dog. In 1845 the Illustrated London News reported on a Newfoundland dog that had repeatedly tried to drown himself: "The dog had been acting less lively than usual for days. However, then it was seen to throw himself in the water and endeavor to sink by preserving perfect stillness of the legs and feet." The story goes on to say that the dog was repeatedly rescued and tied up. However, as soon as the dog was released he entered the water again and tried to sink himself. This occurred several times until at last the dog appeared to tire. The report continues "The animal appeared to get exhausted, and by dint of keeping his head determinedly under water for few minutes, succeeded at last in obtaining his object, for when taken out this time he was indeed dead."

In a more recent story, in 2012 and according to animal rights campaigners' claims, they have witnessed many bears reported to have starved themselves to death to escape their captivity in China and Vietnam. Some bears are kept inside very small cages by the keepers, who harvest their bile, a digestive juice stored in the gall bladder, which is prized in traditional Chinese medicine. An estimated 12,000 bears are kept in captivity; the bile is removed from the bear by inserting a catheter tube through a permanent incision in the abdomen and gall bladder. Sometimes, a permanently implanted metal tube is used. The painful process is generally carried out twice a day. Therefore, many bears were reported to have starved themselves to death, in order to end their misery.

The Stories go on and on about animals of which they indicate an act of suicide. However, some may ask or wonder if animals do have the self-realization or awareness to decide to end their lives and if they do make rational decisions and choices. Well, from a rational point of view, let's think of it this way when a gazelle runs away from a lion's attack, and when the birds seek sanctuary when the rain falls, rational thinking tells us that all creatures have a sense of existence, self-awareness/realization to some degree. When the gazelle or bird runs for safety, that's a survival instinct. When animals decide to end their lives, all they do is just ignore that survival instinct, and that's how they end their lives. On a similar note, sadly when humans decide to end their lives they also ignore their survival instinct and surrender to a reason which they believe is rational or a way out.

Usually social beings, whether humans or animals must surely have a sense of self since they have a sense of their society and their place in it. Many suicides committed under an intense wave of emotions, depression, rage, desperation, panic, love, and for some people, self-suicide is the only way out to avoid social suicide. It makes sense if an animal can have enough instinct to know what would and wouldn't kill it "survival instinct". And that brings us to the notion of animals having a sense of self-awareness and existence, maybe not as humans do, but to a certain extent.

Humans and animals have the same brain. We share the limbic system (the emotion circuit) with most animals, and ours is very similar to other mammals. Also, serotonin regulates the brainstem in mammals, which controls basic functions like eating and sleeping. The irregularity or imbalances in serotonin may lead to depression and anxiety in humans and animals, based on its levels.

How consuming mistreated animals affects us?

As mentioned earlier, the way we treat animals and provide for them makes a significant difference to the quality of products they produce for their consumers. Sadly, it's very rare to find a decent treatment to slaughter animals since big industries took over.

Furthermore, the mistreatment of animals starts from birth, what the animal was fed, how the animal was fed, where the animals spent their time before the slaughter, the transportations of animals, the hygiene environment was provided to animals, the type of environment that was provided to the animals, how the animal is slaughtered or killed, and what follows after that, until the meat or the animal product ends up on your plate.

According to the Journal of Animal Science and researchers at the University of Milan's Faculty of Veterinary Medicine, fear experienced by animals during slaughter significantly elevates levels of stress hormones such as adrenaline, cortisol, and other hormones in the meat. Studies on human consumption of artificial growth hormones, which are believed by many that affect our reproductive systems and other bodily processes, have already resulted in policy changes in many countries, including those that make up the E.U. Attention is now turning to these naturally occurring fear-induced hormones as scientists worry that their consumption causes similar problems.

In addition, such mistreatment and lack of care for these animals lead to severe depression and traumas. I have seen some extremely horrible and horrifying videos were filmed covertly at animal farms, or better call them warehouses. You can clearly see workers hitting the animals, keeping animals or birds in a very small space where many of them die from suffocation. Animals and birds such as chickens and turkeys are transported in small and dirty cages on top of each other where many of them die on the way before reaching their official destiny of death. They also develop many diseases caused by the piles of feces which they live on. I truly urge you to watch a documentary called "Earthlings". See for yourself how these animals were treated by humans (if they are humans) and then decide if you still want to be a part of it.

Often I wonder, do we really expect any nutrition or benefits to come from those poorly fed and mistreated animals? If there is one thing we're getting from them, it is certainly something negative.

Depressed animals and human diseases

It may sound a little strange to some people that traumatized and depressed animals affect humans when consuming them or their products. However, depression is depression whether in humans or in animals – this is based on the limbic system (which is present in humans and animals), as well as the hormones related to behaviors. Depression, in general, doesn't only affect the brain and behavior, but it affects the entire body even on the cellular level. Depression has been linked with other health problems, including cancers and other diseases.

A major depressive episode includes poor moods over an extended period of time, or loss of interest/pleasure - which may be accompanied by symptoms such as weight loss, fatigue, sleep disturbance, and thoughts of suicide. There is strong evidence to suggest that depression is a genetic disorder BDNF and the serotonin transporter genes are two prominent candidate genes. A seminal study, according to US National Library of Medicine, indicates how the serotonin transporter gene can interact with the environment to cause depression. Serotonin is associated with suicide, aggression, and impulsivity, and selective serotonin reuptake inhibitors (SSRIs) are commonly used to treat depression. On the cellular level, glial cells called oligodendrocytes can be reduced in number in individuals with depression and bipolar disorder. A network of brain areas, including the cingulate gyrus, hypothalamus, brainstem, and amygdala, have been associated with depression.

According to Prof. Wayne Drevets and Jonathan Savitz, M.D., this hypothesis in Brain Cells and Depression/Bipolar Disorder indicates that Post-mortem studies of depression have commonly shown that glial cells, called oligodendrocytes, are decreased in number. Glial cells play vital roles in brain function, which include supporting a network of brain systems. Their dysfunction may interfere with a brain circuit involved in maintaining the balance between the normal responses to stressful or anxiety-provoking events. Also, there's an intriguing dynamic exist between serotonin transporters and the environment. Use the Chromosome Map of Disorders and Processes to explore this and other candidate genes. Advances in genomic technology have added considerable power to the search for candidate genes for depression. Ironically, this has led to an increasingly complex picture, which is due to the different forms of the disorder (heterogeneity) and environmental interactions.

In other words, depression and anxiety in animals may get transported to humans in the same way as diseases by consuming the depressed meats and products. Basically, all caged animals are mistreated and depressed. Many food product corporations don't provide the healthy environment to the animals in order to cut costs and aiming for bigger profits. Usually, animals are kept in small enclosures where they sit on each other and on their own feces, especially chickens. And also cattle are usually kept in very small spaces where they can barely stand up. They stand, sit and sleep on their own feces where sometimes the pen is not cleaned for weeks. Many of those big corporations don't provide big enough spaces for their animals in order to fit more stock, and to disable the animals from moving (fewer calories to burn). They feed the animals frequently with less movement so they can become fatter and bigger. The faster the companies get their animals in the market, the faster they make money and the bigger and fatter the animal get, the more money they will make based on the animal's weight.

Animals kept in poor conditions are usually depressed, anxious, afraid, traumatized, sick, frustrated, confused and very tired of living in such conditions. All these traumatic experiences which the animals go through are imprinted in their cells and genes (meats and products). When we consume such meats and products, we also get affected maybe in the same form of depression, anxiety etc. which is already imprinted in the animal products, or maybe in some other form of diseases. Think about the mad cow disease, swine flu, birds flu, and heavens know what's next - but the bottom line is, don't expect to have a peaceful and healthy meal from tortured, depressed and miserable animals. I'm sure there are some other alternatives for better treatments such as "free range/cage free chicken, eggs or animals". However, we should ask ourselves if all the cage-free, kosher and Halal labelled products really meet the criteria of being called caged-free Kosher and Halal.

Halal and Kosher

Halal and Kosher are religious dietary laws that validate the type of foods are allowed to be consumed, as well as how animals should be treated and slaughtered. Halal and Kosher diets aren't practiced only by Muslims and Jews but by many people with different beliefs, especially because of the regularities the animals must undergo before the slaughter.

Halal and Kosher must be done in accordance with established religious practices. An Imam or a Rabbi has to be present, and all the fluid, such as blood in both Halal and kosher meats must be completely drained out and washed. Kosher meat is also salted or washed in salt water to draw out all bodily fluids. Halal meat is usually all cuts of lamb, beef and chicken, where kosher meat, in the case of beef, only use the fore quarter, not hind portions.

As will elaborate more about Halal and kosher diets and their health benefits, such diets seem to be wiser than non-Halal/kosher diets, because of the way the animal must be treated and slaughtered. However, some questions still remain unsatisfyingly answered, such as if all animals which are stamped as Halal and Kosher are really Halal and Kosher! Did those animals really undergo a certain process and has been verified as Halal or Kosher by a trustworthy organization/s without any political or commercial influences? Some questions have always been clouded when it comes to those labels on the food products, and I wonder if these stamps and labels are what they claim to be.

I for one used to follow a Kosher/Halal meat diet, until I stopped eating meat all together back in 2011, for reasons that will be explained in this chapter. And I also would like you, my dear reader, to know that I'm not a religious authority, do not represent one, claim to be nor be or will ever be. I'm just a researcher who brings to you facts and truths to be further examined and thought about. I assure you that what you are reading here is based on extensive researches. The sources or the origins and the authorities of the claims are not my own opinion. In other words "don't shoot the messenger"!

Halal: The very word "Halal" in Arabic means "permissible" according to various dictionaries. The word Halal is often referred to as an action that is permissible to use or engage in according to the Islamic teachings. However, the focus will be only on Halal foods in this segment, and more specifically on Halal meats.

The consumption of pork (swine) is forbidden for Muslims and Jews. For Muslims, it is stated in the Quran in 2:173, 5:3, 6:145 and 16:115. Therefore, there is no Halal or Kosher pork.

According to the Gulf Standard, general requirements for animals and birds slaughtering states: "Slaughter (dabh): Involves cutting of the animal's trachea, esophagus and jugular veins. This method is mostly used in case of sheep, cattle and birds." And "The slaughterer must be Muslim or Kitabi (Jewish, Christian, Mandaean or monotheistic person). " Jews and Christians are usually referred to in Islam as Ahlu Al Kitab "people of the book". Muslims are allowed to eat their meats, and it's considered as Halal as the official documents indicate, as well as the Quran in 5:5. It clearly states: "The food of the People of the Book is lawful unto you and yours is lawful unto them." - Quran in 5:5.

Also, the same document indicates (Quran 5:3) what shouldn't be consumed and is forbidden from eating or is as non-halal:

"Carrion: The animal which dies a natural death and is not slaughtered in due form; the term also applies to any part cut from the body of an animal before it is slaughtered.

Strangled animal: The animals that die from asphyxia.

Fatally beaten animal: The animal that has died as a result of a severe beating by a stick, or any other object, (exception to these are birds or animals shot dead by arrows or bullets with the intention of hunting).

Animals killed by falling from a height: The animal which has died as a result of falling from a height or into a pit or similar hole.

Horn-butted animal: The animal that has died as a result of butting by horns of another animal.

An animal which has been partially devoured by predatory animals: The animal (other than those hunted) which has been partially devoured by predatory animals or birds of prey.

An animal which has been dedicated to anyone else other than God: The animal upon which at the time of slaughter, a name other than that of God was invoked, such as the name of an idol or false deity."

These are the rules for the meat to be labelled as Halal meat, and many people focus more on the religious-legal side of the Halal or Kosher, rather than on the meaning and principal behind it or the hygienic and spiritual side of the Halal and Kosher. For example, the whole meaning of Halal is to guarantee the welfare of the animal by providing as much peace and care before the animal or bird is consumed by humans.

It's believed by Muslims, especially Sufis (a doctrine that focuses more on wisdom, peace and spirituality), the more peace and comfort you provide for the animal or bird, the greater blessings you get out of it when it's consumed. Blessed food is healthy food and it provides the best nutrition and heals from diseases.

Sufis also believe that the animal or bird must be facing the Kaaba in Mecca when it's being slaughtered because of the gravity pull – which is caused by the dynamic energy that is being generated by millions of pilgrims rotating all year round around the Kaaba. The rotation of millions generates a gravitational pull, which will help the blood to be drained out and create a peaceful state for the animal or bird. Also, the knife has to be very sharp and straight. The animal or bird shouldn't feel it when it passes across. Also, if the animal suffers during the slaughter - then, the slaughter won't be considered as Halal. Sufis also believe that the animal or bird shouldn't see the knife before or when it's being slaughtered. Therefore, the slaughterer should always hide the knife behind their back. The method of slaughter should be a very quick, deep stroke across the throat, with a perfectly sharp blade with no nicks or unevenness. This method is also painless, causes unconsciousness within two seconds, and is widely recognized as the most humane method of slaughter possible.

The Sufis also explain why the animal or bird must be dedicated to God only and no other deity, and the name of Allah which is the (Arabic name of God) has to be invoked. This is because they believe when an animal or bird is offered to another deity but God it won't be slaughtered as humanely and will lose its blessings and peace. Therefore, it won't be Halal or blessed - and many diseases and illnesses will follow because the animal or bird died scared or didn't die in a peaceful state.

Kosher:

Kosher (Kashér) means "fit". When it's applied to foods, such as kosher foods, it means the foods are fit or acceptable to be consumed. Kosher foods are those that meet the regulations of kashrut (Jewish dietary law). "Kashrut" comes from the Hebrew root Kaf-Shin-Reish, meaning fit, proper or correct. And food that is not in accordance with Jewish law is called "treif" which originally means "torn". Treif is a similar concept in Islamic tradition for non-halal food "Haram".

Originally, treif derives from a category of non-kosher meat, such as an animal that has been ravaged in the field (terefah) or "torn" (lit. torn, from the commandment not to eat animals that have been torn by other animals), in keeping with prohibition in the Torah (Old testament) in Exodus 22:31. It was later interpreted indicating any animal or fowl that is unfit for consumption due to a defect, disease or inflicted wounds. By extension, the term now applies to all products that are non-kosher. A kosher animal can be treif if improperly slaughtered or found to be diseased or malformed after inspection by a kashrut supervisor.

The word "kosher" can also be used and often is used to describe ritual objects that are made in accordance with Jewish teachings and are fit for ritual use. Lists of some kosher foods are found in the books of Leviticus 11:1-47 and Deuteronomy 14:3-20, as there are also certain kosher rules.

The books of Deuteronomy and Leviticus state, any animal that chews the cud and has a cloven hoof is ritually clean, but animals that only chew the cud or only have cloven hooves are not clean - non-kosher.

However, Kosher slaughtering also has rules as Halal. The mammals and birds must be slaughtered in accordance with Jewish law. In Deuteronomy 12:21 "we may not eat animals that died of natural causes", Deuteronomy 14:21 "or that were killed by other animals". In addition, the animal must have no disease or flaws in the organs at the time of slaughter. These restrictions do not apply to fish; only to the flocks and herds according to the book of Numbers 11:22.

Ritual slaughter is known as Shechitah and the person who performs the slaughter is called a "Shochet", both from the Hebrew root Shin-Cheit-Teit. The method of slaughter is also a quick, deep stroke across the throat with a perfectly sharp blade with no nicks or unevenness. This method similarly as Halal is also painless, causes unconsciousness within two seconds, and is widely recognized as the most humane method of slaughter possible.

Another advantage of Shechitah is to ensure rapid, complete draining of the blood, which is also necessary to render the meat kosher.

The Shochet is not simply a butcher. He must be a pious man, well-trained in Jewish law, particularly as it relates to kashrut. In smaller, more remote communities, the rabbi and the shochet were often the same person.

Draining of blood is also a rule in kosher meat. The Torah prohibits consumption of blood as mentioned in the book of Leviticus 7:26-27 and Leviticus 17:10-14. This is the only dietary law that has a reason specified in Torah: we do not eat blood because the life of the animal (literally, the soul of the animal) is contained in the blood. This applies only to the blood of birds and mammals, not the blood that of fish. Therefore, it is necessary to remove all blood from the flesh of kosher animals.

The first step in this process occurs at the time of slaughter. As discussed above, shechitah allows for rapid draining of most of the blood. The remaining blood must be removed, either by broiling or soaking and salting. The liver may only be kashered by broiling, because it has so much blood in it and such complex blood vessels. This final process must be completed within 72 hours after slaughter and before the meat is frozen or ground. Most butchers and all frozen food vendors take care of the soaking and salting for the consumer.

Also, an egg that contains a blood spot may not be eaten. People who follow the kosher diet are often advised to break an egg into a glass and check it before putting it into a heated pan; otherwise, if a blood-stained egg touches the heated pan, the pan becomes non-kosher. And if the recipe calls for multiple eggs, the eggs should be broken individually into the glass separately, so all the eggs are not wasted if the last one is not kosher!

Fats and Nerves are also forbidden in kosher meat. The sciatic nerve and its adjoining blood vessels may not be eaten. The process of removing this nerve is time-consuming and not cost-effective, so most American kosher slaughterers simply sell the hind quarters to non-kosher butchers. A certain kind of fat, known as chelev, surrounds the vital organs and liver, and may not be eaten. Kosher butchers remove this. Modern scientists have found biochemical differences between this type of fat and the permissible fat around the muscles and under the skin.

Separation of Meat and Dairy in the Kosher diet: on three separate occasions, the Torah says "do not boil a kid in its mother's milk" (a kid means a young goat), as well as the books of Exodus 23:19, Exodus 34:26 and Deuteronomy 14:21. The Oral Torah explains that this passage prohibits eating meat and dairy together. The Rabbis extended this prohibition to include not eating poultry and milk together. In addition, the Talmud prohibits cooking meat and fish together or serving them on the same plate, because it is considered to be unhealthy. It is, however, permissible to eat fish and dairy together, and it is quite common (such as lox and cream cheese). It is also permissible to eat eggs and dairy together.

This separation includes not only the foods themselves but the utensils, pots and pans with which they are cooked, the plates and flatware from which they are eaten, the dishwashers or dishpans in which they are cleaned, the sponges with which they are cleaned and the towels with which they are dried. A kosher household will have at least two sets of pots, pans and dishes: one for meat and one for dairy.

One must wait a significant amount of time between eating meat and dairy. Opinions differ and vary from three to six hours after meat. This is because fatty residues and meat particles tend to cling to the mouth. From dairy to meat, however, one need only rinse his/her mouth and eat a neutral solid, like bread, unless the dairy product in question is also a type that tends to stick in the mouth.

In conclusion, the Halal and Kosher diets are wholesome and respectful to animals, for the animal's well-being as well as for humans. However, I find it hard to believe the sources they stamp Halal and Kosher on their products as trustworthy. There are plenty of trustworthy sources, and there are also plenty of businesses and money driven sources which are certified to label their meats or food products as Halal and Kosher. Unfortunately, this clean diet also became an industry just like any other industry.

In fact, I have seen some covertly filmed videos showing what is really going on inside the animal farming industry including Kosher and Halal. A great example is a documentary called "Earthlings". The documentary contains some horrible leaked footages where clearly can be seen what really happens to the animal, and what the animal goes through before the slaughter – including the so-claimed Kosher and Halal. And for those who still believe that animals don't have feelings or don't feel pain! I guess nothing can convince them and they chose to stay in denial. Or, they can build up some courage and watch this documentary or similar ones, and then decide whether to believe or to shrug their shoulders as nothing happened - "what a wonderful day jolly".

As you've read so far - pain, frustration, fear, depression, sense of helplessness and other unpleasant feelings the animals pass through will also be carried on to the cellular level of that animal. Those feelings will remain, especially the last feeling the animal experiences before its death. Feelings; such as fear and depression, will be imprinted in the memory of that animal. Then, it is passed to its meat, organs and whatever products comes out of it. Those imprinted feelings may also pass to us and we will be affected by them, as we are what we eat.

On a similar note, consuming blood by any form will lead to violence in one's character and the non-halal or kosher meat contains lots of blood because the blood is not properly drained especially if the animal has been shot instead of slaughtered. Also, when the animal is sedated before it is killed, that sedatives will cause numbness in the brain and organs. This leads the animal to die unnaturally in a state of confusion and fear!

Halal, Kosher and the living hell

As I've stated earlier, I used to follow Kosher and Halal diets before I stopped eating meat in early 2011. After I have investigated the "how and what" makes such diet great and healthy, the surprise was semi-expected when I found out that most of these stamps indicating Halal and Kosher are bogus!

Here's why - both diets forbid eating land animals are fed on other land animals (carnivores and omnivores – sea creatures are not included). Only vegetating-herbivores land animals can be Halal and Kosher. Or in simpler terms – only land animals or birds without claws and/or canine teeth. Such as, sheep, beef, chickens, turkey etc. which make up those aren't meat eaters, (not pigs because they have canines and they are meat eater).

Furthermore, based on the environment provided for the animals and birds and especially chickens, most animals and birds nowadays aren't fit to be Halal and Kosher or even otherwise. For example, chickens are on top of each other living on their mountains feces and most of them drop dead from ammoniac asphyxiation and other chemicals which cause their lungs to give up or beg for death. The dead chickens will be lying around for days in the filthy inhumane warehouses where no sunlight or fresh air exist in such hell except some fans which make things worse. The other chickens "semi-zombified" start pecking on other dead chickens which are dead for days. There's clearly something wrong with those chickens to behave in such a way towards their fellow chickens! So, those chickens that peck on and ate even a small bit of a dead chicken, are they considered Halal and Kosher? Impossible! All elements and requirements for both diets don't exist in such environment. The rituals and a sharp knife etc. do not matter anymore for a chicken is begging for any death other than this hell. If a chicken is psychologically and physically unstable and was consumed by a human, what would be the physical and psychological effect on the human? The effect will be many things but healthy isn't one of them.

The Chicken Industry

Almost all chickens are raised for their meat, or as referred to by the meat industry "broiler chickens". They spend their lives in overcrowded and massive windowless sheds where the sun and fresh air has no place in there and these sheds typically hold as many as 40,000 birds. We know that chickens are social birds and can function well in groups, but not in crowded groups of thousands in the same sunless and airless shed. However, no such social order is possible in these sheds and in their frustration they ruthlessly peck at each other, causing injuries and deaths. The extremely overcrowded sheds on the farms also result in extreme filth and horrible diseases, which you will never see or hear about based on the secrecy of those places. And don't be so naïve to think that "but my government won't allow that" because your government is allowing it whether directly or indirectly! These chicken sheds are full of the smell of ammonia from the chicken's feces and sweat and the air ventilation fans make the problem even worse. The chickens are forced to smell and live in these horrible conditions for as long as they are alive or better say "semi-alive or zombified". This causes many chickens to suffer from chronic respiratory diseases, weakened immune systems, bronchitis, and "ammonia burn," a painful eye condition, as well as ammonia burn that is clearly visible on every chicken that I see at any supermarket till this very day.

Ammonia burns are painful burns. Patches can be found on the chicken feet, stomach, legs, or wherever the chicken spent most of its time laying around in that small closure. Those painful burns are caused by the chicken's feces, where the chickens spend most of their life time sitting on, and it burns because it's acidic based. However, there's a very sly and dirty trick performed by the butchers - and that is the removal of those ammonia burn patches before packing the chicken and then placing them in fridges. This trick is just to hide the painful history of that chicken, and what it passed through before it was packaged. The removal of patches is very visible when you see skin removed from the stomach or the feet etc. You can check online for images what the burns look like, it's called "ammonia burns".

In addition, a 2010 study by the Consumer Reports found, a shocking 83 percent of grocery market chickens tested were infected with either campylobacter or salmonella bacteria or even both. The extremely high occurrence of dangerous contaminants in chicken flesh is largely due to the filthy conditions in the sheds where they are raised. On factory farms, they are fed large quantities of powerful antibiotics to keep them alive in conditions that would otherwise kill them. Chickens are given nearly four times the amount of antibiotics as humans or cattle in the United States.

Chickens are also genetically enhanced and regularly dosed with drugs to make them grow faster and larger. The average breast of an 8-week-old chicken is seven times heavier today than it was 25 years ago. Because of this unnaturally accelerated weight gain, these very young birds frequently die of heart attacks and lungs collapses. Something like that would almost never happen in nature. According to Feedstuffs, a meat-industry magazine, "Broilers now grow so rapidly that the heart and lungs are not developed well enough to support the remainder of the body, resulting in congestive heart failure and tremendous death losses."

Consequently, chickens on today's factory farm always become crippled because their legs cannot support the weight of their bodies. In fact, by the age of 6 weeks, 90 percent of broiler chickens are morbidly obese and can no longer walk. Many crippled chickens on factory farms die when they can no longer walk to reach the water nozzles.

When birds are very young (usually just 1 to 10 days old) hot blades are used to cut large chunks off their sensitive beaks so they won't peck each other out of frustration - caused by the intensely crowded conditions. Sometimes their toes, spurs, and combs are also cut off. The birds are not given any painkillers to ease the agony of this mutilation, and much de-beaked (their beaks cut off) chickens starve to death because they are in too much pain to eat. I can't agree any less with Dr. Joy Mench, a poultry scientist at the University of California, she said "gallus neglectedus" or "neglected chicken," because their welfare is completely ignored.

There's no positive benefits what-so-ever for your health from such abused animals. According to a major 2006 Harvard study of 135,000 people, those who frequently ate grilled, skinless chicken had a 52 percent higher chance of developing bladder cancer than those who didn't.

The biggest shock is, many of those chickens are labeled as Halal and Kosher. I don't see where the peace and comforts are for the animals' welfare in such treatments before the slaughter! On the contrary, I can only see the welfare and comfort of the Halal and Kosher industry pockets. The Karma is also paid by the consumer as a Harvard study shows. Although, chickens are the most abused but this also happens to cattle and other animals.

Once again, I'm not raising an alarm against all the Halal and Kosher labels and organizations, nor on every deli or butcher. I believe that there are still some good breeders and farmers out there who believe in giving good welfare to their animals. I also believe and have witnessed some free-range chickens farms where chickens freely live on an open land and lay their eggs freely. Also cattle breeders with their own cows running freely and vegetating on a green landscape, and are providing the best milk and products. There aren't many but they do exist. And if you have decided to eat meat and consume other animal products, you better do your homework before feeding yourself and your family something that was heinously bred, lived and killed.

"The greatness of a nation can be judged by the way its animals are treated."

- Mahatma Gandhi

"He who is cruel to animals becomes hard also in his dealings with men. We can judge the heart of a man by his treatment of animals."

- Immanuel Kant

"The time is always right to do what is right."

- Martin Luther King, Jr

Chapter 11
The Plastic Age

There is a three-age system in archaeology and physical anthropology, these are the periodization of human prehistory and history into three consecutive time periods, named for their respective tool-making technologies.

First, we had the Stone Age and its period lasted roughly 3.4 million years and ended between 6000 BC and 2000 BC. The second age was the Bronze Age, estimated around 3200 – 600 BC. Then, the Iron Age, around 1200 BC. Furthermore, we can consider the age we live in now as the forth age – and metaphorically call it the "Plastic Age".

In the 1920s, the Plastic Age was progressing rapidly and started to dominate the era during the 1960s. Now, plastics are everywhere. While you're reading this book, there are numerous of plastic objects within your reach (your computer, your pen, your phone etc.). Plastic is any material that can be shaped or molded into any form, and most of it is man-made.

Furthermore, plastics are made from petroleum. According to the American Chemistry Council, petroleum is a carbon-rich raw material, and plastics are large carbon-containing compounds. They are large molecules called polymers, which are composed of repeating units of shorter carbon-containing compounds called monomers. Chemists combine various types of monomers in many different arrangements to make an almost infinite variety of plastics with different chemical properties. Most plastics are chemically inert and will not react chemically with other substances. You can store alcohol, soap, water, gasoline and even acid in a plastic container without dissolving the container itself. And since plastic can be molded into almost an infinite variety of shapes, you can find it in toys, cups, bottles, utensils, wiring, cars, even in bubble gum. Plastic has revolutionized the world.

However, because plastic doesn't react chemically with most other substances, and doesn't dissolve even in acid (you can store acid in plastic containers), therefore, plastic disposal poses a difficult and significant environmental problem. Plastics remain in the environment for centuries. Consequently, plastic is already causing major problems for humans and the environment. Some new technologies are being developed to make plastic from biological substances like corn oil. These types of plastics might be biodegradable and better for the environment, as well as for humans.

The risk of plastic in general

Plastic water and beverage bottles, as well as plastic food containers, have become an essential component of the modern era the "Plastic Age". However, foods and drinks stored and packaged in plastic products aren't so healthy after all, and many people aren't aware of the risks. Most plastics are made from petroleum (oil or natural gas) - plastic contain a whole host of other chemicals (which are never labeled), the chemicals can be toxic to humans and the environment in general.

In the last few decades, humans have managed to dump tons of garbage into the ocean. And since plastic takes thousands of years to decay, plastic has become one major and devastating problems to our echo-system. As a result, fish and wildlife are becoming contaminated. In addition, the toxins contained in plastics have also become a major threat to our health and other species since the toxins have infiltrated our food-chain.

In the most polluted places in the ocean, the masses of plastic have exceeded the amount of plankton (organisms provide a crucial source of nutrients to many large fish and whales). According to the Sea Education Society, scientists studied plastics in the Atlantic and estimated - there are 580,000 pieces of plastic per a square kilometer, and this is only in the Atlantic Ocean.

According to the National Geographic Society, plastics spread throughout the ocean; Styrofoam breaks into smaller parts, polystyrene components and it sinks lower in the ocean, and as a result, the pollutant spreads throughout the sea.

In fact, not only do the toxins in plastic affect the ocean, they also act like sponges, soaking up other toxins from outside sources before entering the ocean again. As these chemicals are ingested by animals in the ocean, humans as well will ingest contaminated fish and other sea-foods.

According to the Ecology Center in Berkley California, dangers of plastic to humans can occur through direct toxicity from lead, cadmium, and mercury. These toxins are dangerous to humans and have been found in fish in the ocean. Diethylhexyl phthalate (DEHP) contained in some plastics, is a toxic carcinogen. Other toxins in plastics are directly linked to cancers, birth defects, immune system problems, and childhood developmental issues. Other types of toxic plastics are BPA or health-bisphenol-A, along with phthalates. Both of these are of great concern to human health. BPA can be found in many things including plastic bottles and food packaging materials. Over time the polymer chains of BPA breaks down and can enter the human body in many ways, from drinking contaminated water to eating fish exposed to the broken down toxins. BPA is a known chemical that interferes with human hormonal function.

The terrifying effect of plastic on human health

Dr. Frederick Vom Saal, a Professor of Biological Sciences, University of Missouri and a leading researcher in the field of developmental biology, stated, just this one chemical Bisphenol-A which is used to make hard clear plastics called polycarbonate, is produced at over 7 billion pounds a year, and as it is a non-recyclable plastic, what's happening to it? It's been thrown away into the environment! The evidence from Europe, Asia, and United States is that every person examined has these chemicals in their bodies. There's a study in Japan where women with elevated levels of Bisphenol-A were the women who were rapidly miss-carrying, and are now never able to have a successful pregnancy. When you go out into the ocean, you see that the ocean is full of these plastic products.

Researchers have found, there are three kinds of plastics have been shown to leach or release some dangerous toxic chemicals when heated, worn or put under pressure: polycarbonate - which leaches bisphenol A, polystyrene - which leaches styrene, and PVC or polyvinyl chloride - which breaks down into vinyl chloride and sometimes contains phthalates which essentially can leach.

Nowadays, almost all water bottles and food products are packed, wrapped or stored in plastic containers, bottled or sealed by plastic. Plastic is the environment's worst nightmare and will take a very long time for nature to get rid of it. Therefore we recycle it over and over, and by doing so we think that we've solved the environmental issue, but the reality is we're still too far from solving it. The Great Pacific garbage patch, also known as the Pacific Trash Vortex is an evidence that we are abusing the environment with our trash and plastic wastage. According to NOAA (The National Oceanic and Atmospheric Administration), 90% of the trash found there was plastic, 80% of the plastic in the ocean comes from land sources, while 20%

comes from ships at sea. In other words, most of those trash islands are plastic, objects of plastic origins, or contain plastic debris. The Great Pacific garbage patch is located within the North Pacific Gyre (135°W to 155°W and 35°N and 42°N), keep in mind that this is only one of five major oceanic gyres, and there are other major garbage or trash islands in the oceans, like the one is the Sargasso Sea and others.

What are the health risks in recycling plastics?

There is a coding system that is used on plastic bottles, containers and products. There's usually a number inside the recycling logo to identify the type of plastic it is made of. The symbols used in the codes contain arrows that cycle clockwise to form a triangle and circling a number, often with a number (1 – 7) which is the code representing the type of plastic below the triangle.

PETE	HDPE	V	LDPE	PP	PS	OTHER
Polyethylene Terephthalate	High Density Polyethylene	Vinyl	Low Density Polyethylene	Polypropylene	Polystyrene	Other
soda bottles	milk, water and juice jugs	clear food packaging	bread bags	ketchup bottles	meat trays	ketchup
water bottles		shampoo bottles	frozen food bags	yogurt and margarine tubs	egg cartons	3 & 5 gallon water bottles
shampoo bottles	detergent bottles		squeezable bottles (mustard, honey)		cups and plates	some juice bottles
mouthwash bottles	yogurt and margarine tubs					
peanut butter jars	grocery bags					

The water bottles we buy at supermarkets, corner stores or vending machines are made of a lightweight plastic called PET or code 1. According to researchers at Johann Wolfgang Goethe University in Frankfurt, Germany, the bottles made from a type of plastic known as PET, for polyethylene terephthalate code 1, the water that is contained in those bottles may also pack a substantial quantity of estrogen (female sex hormones).

A recent study at the Yale School of Medicine, published in The Endocrine Society journal, Hormones and Cancer, found the exposure in the womb to chemicals such as Bisphenol-A (BPA) can increase the risk of breast cancer. BPA belongs to a group of chemicals called xenoestrogens, which are used to make pesticides, herbicides and plastics. Xenoestrogens act as estrogen in the body, attaching themselves to estrogen receptors in both males and females.

These artificial estrogens can interfere with normal hormonal signaling. We should take measures to avoid these hormone-mimicking chemicals as they may increase the risk of breast, prostate and reproductive cancers, reduce fertility and immune function, cause early puberty in children, menstrual irregularities and other disorders. However, xenoestrogens, BPA has the greatest impact on our health. BPA is used to make hard, clear plastic containers for items such as baby bottles, water bottles, microwave ovenware, eating utensils, milk and juice containers, as well as the plastic coating inside metal cans.

Moreover, the increase of estrogen in males and females causes very serious problems and health issues. Estrogen is already found in all men, and women do need small amounts of testosterone (male hormone). Nevertheless, there is a growing need to understand the effects of estrogen in men. Like all hormones, estrogen needs to be kept in balance in both men and women. Chronic health conditions are more likely to occur in men as a result of estrogen levels becoming too high.

The risk of high estrogen in males

Estrogen is a female hormone which belongs to a set of molecules known as steroid hormones. It is produced in the ovaries of women and small amounts are made in the testes, adrenal and pituitary glands in males. Men usually have low levels of estrogen and a number of undesirable symptoms can occur when levels of estrogen are too high. Measures should be taken to lower estrogen levels if it is too high in men.

Studies shows, some very serious problems may occur when the estrogen levels increase in males such as:

Gynecomastia/Male breast growth is the growth of male breasts.

Low sex drive: occur to men with high levels of estrogen may experience a problem known as erectile dysfunction – the inability to maintain an erection.

Infertility: it is determined by the amount of sperms a male may produce, as well as the movement of the sperm and whether they can survive long enough to reach and fertilize an egg. Men with high exposure to estrogen have a higher rate of infertility than men with less exposure - simply because estrogen lowers the sperm's mobility.

Stroke risk: excess estrogen may cause blood clots. Men with higher levels of estrogen may be at higher risks of having a stroke.

Heart attack: when men get older they produce less testosterone. This causes hormonal imbalances with estrogen becoming more dominant than testosterone. Such imbalances are often overlooked as a possible cause of heart disease.

Prostate problems: some studies show, excess estrogen may cause prostate cancer, but once cancer occurs, the estrogen may have some anticancer effects.

Weight gain: high estrogen levels in men can cause weight gain. In addition, weight gain may also cause higher levels of estrogen. Each issue is related to the other.

Moreover, there is another risk you may not have heard of before and it is somewhat strange and frightening to men. Men with a high level of estrogen may also get male breast cancer! Yes, even men can get male breast cancer. According to a recent article posted on the Food and Drug Administration FDA website. The article was last updated on June 27, 2014, titled "Breast Cancer—Men Get It Too". The article stated, it's a rare condition and around 2000 men are diagnosed with male breast cancer every year but it also states that it is a matter of concern. Therefore, I wanted to share this article with you in this segment as it is from its original source. You can easily find it on

http://www.fda.gov/ForConsumers/ConsumerUpdates/ucm402937.htm

The FDA Article

"Breast Cancer—Men Get It Too

Breast cancer is a disease usually associated with women, as reflected by pink ribbons and gear, but men get it too, albeit rarely.

Because male breast cancer is rare, the Food and Drug Administration (FDA) doesn't have very good clinical trial data on treatments. "We tend to treat men the same way we treat women," says Tatiana M. Prowell, MD, a medical oncologist and breast cancer scientific lead at FDA's Office of Hematology & Oncology Products.

"Men have historically been excluded from breast cancer trials," she adds. "We are actively encouraging drug companies to include men in all breast cancer trials unless there is a valid scientific reason not to. The number of men in breast cancer trials will still be small because male breast cancer is a rare condition, but any information to help men facing this disease is better than none."

Men vs. Women

Each year, about 2,000 cases of male breast cancer (1% of all cases) are diagnosed in the United States, resulting in fewer than 500 deaths, according to the National Cancer Institute. Although it can strike at any age, the disease is usually diagnosed in men 5 to 10 years older than in women and is found most often among men ages 60 to 70.

Prowell says one reason for the late-age (and later stage) diagnosis may be that men don't think of themselves as being at risk of breast cancer. "You'd think that because men have smaller breasts they would notice a lump instantly," Prowell says. "But men don't expect a breast lump to be cancer, whereas most women who feel a breast lump immediately assume the worst."

Most men with breast cancer have painless lumps they can feel. The lumps can develop anywhere on the breast but often are underneath the nipple and areola complex—right in the center. Because men don't have regular mammograms, their breast cancer is usually discovered when they feel sore, such as from a fall or injury.

"Men often attribute breast lumps to some sort of injury. The mass was already there, but they didn't notice it until it got sore," Prowell says.

Men and women share some similar risk factors for breast cancer: high levels of estrogen exposure, a family history of the disease and a history of radiation to the chest. Although all men have estrogen in their bodies, obesity, cirrhosis (liver disease) and Klinefelter's syndrome (a genetic disorder), increase estrogen levels. All are known risk factors for male breast cancer.

If a first-degree relative—their mother, father, brother, sister, children—has breast cancer, men are also at a slight risk to develop the disease themselves. Men who have a BRCA mutation (a mutation or change in a gene that predisposes them to breast cancer) are at a greater risk. While their chance of developing breast cancer is still low (only about 5% to 6%), men with a mutation in BRCA2 have a 100-fold greater risk of developing breast cancer than men in the general population.

"In men and women, having a tumor with estrogen and progesterone hormone receptors is more common than not—but that appears to be even truer in men," Prowell adds.

Treating Male Breast Cancer

Treatment options for men are similar to women's: mastectomy (surgery to remove the breast) or in some cases lumpectomy, radiation, chemotherapy, targeted therapies and hormone therapy.

"Our data on treatments for men are largely based on trials that were conducted in women, or they are retrospective data from a collection of men who were treated over a period of time. We don't have large randomized trials or high-level evidence for treatment of breast cancer in men as we do for women," Prowell says.

Hormonal drug treatments include tamoxifen, a selective estrogen receptor modulator (SERM) that inhibits estrogen receptors, and aromatase inhibitors, which block the production of estrogen from androgens such as testosterone.

"For postmenopausal women, we preferentially use aromatase inhibitors as a first-line treatment for early stage breast cancer and regard tamoxifen as an alternative. It's the opposite for men because what data we have suggest that aromatase inhibitors don't work as well in men. So for men, aromatase inhibitors are usually an alternative or second-line treatment, after tamoxifen," Prowell says.

For men with larger tumors, positive lymph nodes or cancer that has spread, chemotherapy is often recommended in addition to hormonal treatment, just as it is for women. And men with tumors that are HER2-positive are recommended to receive treatment with trastuzumab, an antibody that targets HER2, just as women are.

Genetic Counselling Is a Must

All men with breast cancer should be referred for genetic counselling, Prowell advises.

That's another difference from women, who are not automatically referred to a genetic counsellor for genetic testing, such as for mutations in BRCA-1 or 2. These "tumor suppressor genes" allow breast and other types of cancer to develop when they fail to function normally. Only women with a significant family history or certain other characteristics, such as being young or having triple-negative breast cancer (which don't have estrogen, progesterone or HER2 receptors), are recommended to have genetic testing.

Even among men, there are differences. African American men are more likely than white men to have advanced stage tumors at diagnosis and to develop triple-negative cancers. Their types of tumors are more likely to recur and have fewer treatment options.

People should tell their health care provider if any man in their family has had breast cancer. Prowell says. "Even if your grandfather is deceased, if he had breast cancer, that's important for your health care provider to know. Because male breast cancer is so rare, seeing just one man in a family lineage raises concerns about hereditary breast cancer."

This article appears on FDA's Consumer Updates page, which features the latest on all FDA-regulated products.

June 27, 2014" (*End of the article*).

These are some of the major problems related to high level of estrogen in men, and also estrogen in men may change the appearance of men, as it is common these days to see men with love handles, a wider pelvis, bigger stomach, breast growth (which may be the reason for developing male breast cancer and surely the terrifying increase of prostate cancer among men worldwide).

The risk of high estrogen in females

As previously mentioned, estrogen is the primary female sex hormone as testosterone is to males. Estrogens are a group of compounds named for their importance in both menstrual and oestrous reproductive cycles. It is common for estrogen levels in women to fluctuate widely throughout the menstrual cycle, menopause and pregnancy. However, according to the National Center for Biotechnology Information, U.S. National Library of Medicine, estrogen can rise up to 100 times higher in women during pregnancy. Some side effects of high estrogen levels beside the psychological effects are thyroid dysfunction, weight gain, low sex drive, fluid retention and breast cancer.

In addition, "Estrogen Dominance Syndrome", according to Dr. Ronald Hoffman, "We live in an estrogenic or feminizing environment. Xenoestrogens, such as PCBs, phthalates, pesticides and DDT, cause estrogenic effects. Although banned in 1972, DDT, like its breakdown product DDE, is a xenoestrogen, which is still present in the environment. Chlorine and hormone residues in meats and dairy products can also have estrogenic effects. In men, the estrogenic environment may result in declining quality of sperm or fertility rates.

In women, it may lead to an epidemic of female diseases, all traceable to excess estrogen/deficient progesterone. It is critical to incorporate a pure, clean diet consisting of organic foods whenever possible, in an effort to decrease exposure to harmful xenoestrogens".

What is Xenoestrogen?

Pronounced Zee-no-estrogen, according to Prof. Cheryl S. Watson, Yow-Jiun Jeng, Jutatip Guptarak, The Journal of Steroid Biochemistry and Molecular Biology, V127, xenoestrogens is foreign estrogen mimicker comes a large group (tens of thousands) of foreign compounds derived from synthetic materials pass into our environment through pesticides, herbicides, fungicides, plastics, fuels, car exhausts, dry cleaning chemicals, make-up/cosmetic materials, industrial waste, animal meats which have been fattened with estrogenic drugs, antibiotics, food supplies and countless of other household and personal products which many of us use every day such as makeup products, lotion products and plastic in general.

The effect of Xenoestrogens has been associated with a variety of health issues. In the past ten years, many scientific studies have found solid evidence of adverse effects on human and animal health related to Xenoestrogens. Also, because xenoestrogens have the ability to disturb our natural hormonal systems, which can possibly lead to conditions such as prostate enlargement, prostate cancer, erectile dysfunction, breast cancer, perimenopause (PMS) and menopause, as well as weight gain especially in the abdominal area.

The relation between xenoestrogens and weight gain is these xenoestrogens are fat soluble. In other words, they must find a home to host them. The greater chance is they will find their home within our fat cells. Once they reside within the fat cells it will be difficult to get rid of them.

According to a research presented in the American Journal of Physiology, xenoestrogens have the potential to create an enhanced environment for our bodies to store fat, while making it extremely difficult to lose it.

Another publication based on a group of Japanese researchers who published a study in the Journal of Lipid (fat) Research indicate a common synthetic (men-made) estrogen called bisphenol-A (BPA) which is commonly found in drinking water bottles as well as the coating in metal cans such as food cans and other plastic food containers, both triggers and stimulates two major processes. Besides the increase and storage of body fat which is increasing the number of fat cells (hyperplasia), and enhancing their fat storage abilities to store fat (fat cell hypertrophy).

A research has shown that BPA can leach into foods and beverages from containers contain BPA. Exposure to BPA is a concern because of the possible health effects of BPA on the brain, behavior and prostate gland of fetuses, infants and children. In fact, researchers from Stanford University School of Medicine accidentally discovered that the polycarbonate lab flasks they were using to sterilize the water used in their experiments contained enough BPA to cause hormone-sensitive breast cancer cells to proliferate.

Moreover, there is a research presented in May 2004 in the Journal of Applied Toxicology, xenoestrogens commonly found in many body-care and cosmetic products in the form of p-hydroxybenzoic acid esters or parabens, have been detected in human breast tumor's tissue. This indicates that they are absorbed through the skin.

The National Institute of Environmental Health Sciences, National Institutes of Health, advises against microwaving polycarbonate plastics or cleaning them in the dishwasher, because the plastic may break down over time and allow BPA to leach into foods. Furthermore, we must avoid exposing plastic to any kind of heat especially water bottles. For example, when you buy water or drink in plastic bottles, keep in mind that this bottle was exposed to a degree of heat while the water or drink was in it during delivery, storage, as well as the exposure to the sun heat. I have personally seen supermarkets and stores leave palates of bottles in the sun-heat outside/loading docks in hot weather where the bottles become exposed and overheated by the sunlight. Later, the bottles will be moved to storage rooms or straight into the refrigerators. Plastic bottles full of BPA toxins expand due to heat and leach all kinds of toxins into the water or drinks. That may cause all sorts of hormonal imbalances, cancers and diseases.

This chart describes the plastic, its use, and the possible health effects based on the research of the Ecology Center and other research institutes and organizations:

Plastic	Common Uses	Adverse Health Effects
Polyvinylchloride (#3PVC)	Food packaging, plastic wrap, containers for toiletries, cosmetics, crib bumpers, floor tiles, pacifiers, shower curtains, toys, water pipes, garden hoses, auto upholstery, inflatable swimming pools	Can cause cancer, birth defects, genetic changes, chronic bronchitis, ulcers, skin diseases, deafness, vision failure, indigestion, and liver dysfunction
Phthalates	Softened vinyl products	Endocrine disruption,

Plastic	Common Uses	Adverse Health Effects
(DEHP, DINP, and others)	manufactured with phthalates include vinyl clothing, emulsion paint, footwear, printing inks, non-mouthing toys and children's products, product packaging and food wrap, vinyl flooring, blood bags and tubing, IV containers and components, surgical gloves, breathing tubes, general purpose lab-ware, inhalation masks, many other medical devices	linked to asthma, developmental and reproductive effects. Medical waste with PVC and phthalates is regularly incinerated causing public health effects from the release of dioxins and mercury, including cancer, birth defects, hormonal changes, declining sperm counts, infertility, endometriosis, and immune system impairment.
Polycarbonate, with Bisphenol A (#7)	Water bottles	Scientists have linked very low doses of bisphenol An exposure to cancers, impaired immune function, early onset of puberty, obesity, diabetes, and hyperactivity, among other problems (Environment California)

Plastic	Common Uses	Adverse Health Effects
Polystyrene	Many food containers for meats, fish, cheeses, yogurt, foam and clear clamshell containers, foam and rigid plates, clear bakery containers, packaging "peanuts", foam packaging, audio cassette housings, CD cases, disposable cutlery, building insulation, flotation devices, ice buckets, wall tile, paints, serving trays, throw-away hot drink cups, toys	Can irritate eyes, nose and throat and can cause dizziness and unconsciousness. Migrates into food and stores in body fat. Elevated rates of lymphatic and hematopoietic cancers for workers.
Polyethelyne (#1 PET)	Water and soda bottles, carpet fiber, chewing gum, coffee stirrers, drinking glasses, food containers and wrappers, heat-sealed plastic packaging, kitchenware, plastic bags, squeeze bottles, toys	Suspected human carcinogen

Plastic	Common Uses	Adverse Health Effects
Polyester	Bedding, clothing, disposable diapers, food packaging, tampons, upholstery	Can cause eye and respiratory-tract irritation and acute skin rashes
Urea-formaldehyde	Particle board, plywood, building insulation, fabric finishes	Formaldehyde is a suspected carcinogen and has been shown to cause birth defects and genetic changes. Inhaling formaldehyde can cause cough, swelling of the throat, watery eyes, breathing problems, headaches, rashes, tiredness
Polyurethane Foam	Cushions, mattresses, pillows	Bronchitis, coughing, skin and eye problems. Can release toluene diisocyanate which can produce severe lung problems
Acrylic	Clothing, blankets, carpets made from acrylic fibers, adhesives, contact lenses, dentures, floor	Can cause breathing difficulties, vomiting, diarrhoea, nausea, weakness, headache and

Plastic	Common Uses	Adverse Health Effects
	waxes, food preparation equipment, disposable diapers, sanitary napkins, paints	fatigue
Tetrafluoro-ethelyne	Non-stick coating on cookware, clothes irons, ironing board covers, plumbing and tools	Can irritate eyes, nose and throat and can cause breathing difficulties

Recommendations:

Nowadays, it is difficult to avoid the exposure to xenoestrogens and BPA. However, we can take few simple steps to reduce the overexposure to these disrupting harmful chemicals.

- Buy foods in glass or metal containers
- Avoid heating food in plastic containers, or storing fatty foods in plastic containers or plastic wraps
- Do not give young children plastic teethers or toys especially unmarked or unsafe plastic milk bottles
- Use natural fiber clothing, bedding and furniture
- Avoid all PVC and Styrene products
- Look for products labeled as BPA-free. If a product isn't labeled, keep in mind that some but not all plastics marked with recycle codes 3 or 7 are may be made with BPA.
- Reduce your use of canned foods since most cans are lined with BPA-containing resin.

- Avoid heated plastic. The National Institute of Environmental Health Sciences, National Institutes of Health, advises against microwaving polycarbonate plastics or putting them in the dishwasher, because the plastic may break down over time and allow BPA to leach into the foods.
- Use alternatives - such as glass, porcelain or stainless steel containers for hot foods and liquids instead of plastic containers and utensils.

"Earth provides enough to satisfy every man's needs, but not every man's greed."

- Mahatma Gandhi

"If you really think the environment is less important than the economy, try holding your breath while you count your money."

- Guy McPherson

Chapter 12
Media & Psychology

The psychological factors play an important role in weight loss, gain, obesity as well as our health in general. It is often ignored when people embark on a weight reducing diet, simply because people think the matter is only physical and genetic.

Furthermore, obesity is as much psychological as a physical problem. In addition, numerous considerable researches have shown that the media contribute to the development of obesity. There are various mechanisms have been used by the media which most of them are not known to the general public such as, hypnotic suggestion and Neuro Linguistic Programming NLP techniques. Also, screen time may displace more physical activities, advertising of junk food and fast food increases children's requests for those particular foods and products, snacking increases while watching TV or movies, and late-night screen time may interfere with getting sufficient amounts of sleep, which is a known risk factor for obesity.

As a result, time spent on TV or the majority of commercialized media outlets result in obesity. Contrary to popular opinion, overweight and obesity probably result from small, incremental increases in caloric intake (or increases in sedentary activities). For example, an excess intake of 50 kcal/day (e.g. an extra pat of butter) produces a weight gain of 5 lb/year. Drinking a can of soda per day produces a weight gain of 15 lb/year. As you know already by now, nearly 40% of children's caloric intake comes from solid fat, added sugars, and soda or fruit drinks provide nearly 10% of total calories. Because primarily obesity is caused by an imbalance between energy intake and energy expenditure, as well as screen time may contribute in several different ways.

The influence

Food and beverage advertisements are frequently being broadcast during children's television programming, and much of the foods being advertised are addictive, junk/fast foods or foods of no nutritional values. The main objective of any media advertisement is getting the viewers' attention. Product placement is the paid presence of branded products in movies and is proving to be a potent and influential source of advertising. At a time when the viewers are watching and usually in a trance of watching a movie or a show, an advert will be played in the background (if it's subliminal) or during a commercial break which makes it also effective in terms of conscious branding or "anchoring".

On a related note, anchoring is a Neuro Linguistic Programming (NLP) and Hypnotic term which we also teach at our institute (The MindTech Institute).

An Anchor or in psychology it's called "Focalism", simply defined as a trigger. When it's triggered, it activates a response on the subconscious level, leading to the behavior of what it is installed on. In other words, an anchor is like a program can be installed in the mind – in order to activate this program, it's usually attached to a trigger. The trigger can be a thought, behavior, state, emotion and others. For example, the smell of a specific perfume reminds you of a person, a place or an event etc. Simply, this is an anchor, which is a program in your mind and was established at a time you smelled it where one or more of your senses were active intensely. Another example, you're listening to the radio and a song comes up. The song may remind you of a person, that's because the song is anchored (connected or wired in your mind) by associating that certain person to it.

Also, another good and simple example - if you were to imagine now a juicy lemon, imagine you cut the lemon in half and now you're liking the half you just cut. You're noticing now the feeling of the citric sourness and bitterness of the juicy lemon tingling on your tongue. Although, I'm assuming you don't have a juicy lemon in your hand right now and just licked it, but you certainly have it in your mind with a full experience of the taste and feelings are associated with it. Simply, that's because your subconscious mind already had saved the memory (information) of the taste, feeling, smell, image and maybe some sounds of a lemon from previous experience, and I just fired (activated) that experience or anchor now. I also used another technique called "eliciting sub-modalities" to further enhance the experience. You can learn all that and more during our live or online Neuro Linguistic Programming NLP and Hypnosis Training.

The mind usually saves information and whatever the information are associated with - such as events and experiences through a complex of neuro-wiring and by connecting our senses to networks of various anchors. Such powerful techniques can be easily applied in marketing and can be used unethically sometimes especially by the media.

For instance, here is a very simple example of how junk burger brands apply anchors in their advertisements to anchor children to their brands. Firstly, children like to watch TV, movies etc. The media (movies) produce superhero characters, children like superheroes because they are already being conditioned as they need superheroes to protect them or to become superheroes like them. Junk burger brands use those superhero characters in their junk meals as toys and use slogans such as love it, happy package, we care etc. (positive suggestions leading to anchors). The child now wants to go to those brand restaurants and get the "happy package and a superhero toy" and of course to eat there. The child is already being psychologically programmed - as this place (the restaurant) is a happy place, toys are given, birthdays are celebrated and many colors are present there. The other luring trick is the addiction to the taste which is a "Gustatory (taste) Anchor". By now, the child is already anchored visually and emotionally to the place and brand. Furthermore, they also anchored the child's olfactory and gustatory senses (smell and taste) to the junk burger itself in a form of addiction to the salt, sugar, fat and many other addictive substances. The addictive meal usually is junk burger, meal and the dessert.

To further analyze what's behind this meal - the program is the junk burger/restaurant. The anchors included here are visual such as the logo/media/toy/. Gustatory anchors such as the addictive taste. Olfactory anchor such as the smell of the burger and fries. A kinesthetic anchor such as feeling/happy/superhero. And auditory anchor is the sound/tone/ commercial music of the junk restaurant. The result is; five anchors, one program and billions of victims. This is just one example of food anchoring and marketing. Who are we supposed to blame here, ourselves or the media? The answer is not to waste time and energy on blaming. We just need to educate ourselves more to protect ourselves and spread the message to also protect others!

Other related factors

The biological factor: the human body is made of some 50 trillion to 100 trillion cells. Each cell in the human body contains about 25,000 to 35,000 genes. Genes carry the information that determines our behaviors, which are features or characteristics passed on to us – as we inherited from our parents - all the way back to our ancestors many generations ago. In addition, we are most likely also carrying some of their memories and habits including survival instincts.

According to the U.S. National Library of Medicine, Genetics Home Reference, most people have 23 pairs of chromosomes for a total of 46. One of each pair comes from the mother and the other from the father. This is why we are 50% related to our mothers and 50% to our fathers - and our mothers and fathers carry their parents' DNA and our grandparents also carry their parents' DNA and so on. That would take us back to our ancestors who used to be hunter-gatherers. Therefore, we've inherited some of their behaviors through genes (such as our survival instincts) and we've learnt how to store food to survive. That may explain some overweight cases, for example, people who store more carbohydrates in their bodies, maybe because they are still carrying some dominant genes from their ancestors who were hunters and gatherers and needed to store extra carbohydrates in their bodies to allow them to have more energy to carry on their daily survival tasks. Essentially, their habit of "storing" maybe is still active in a form of "genetic memory".

We have also developed a greedy stomach, many of us tend to eat everything they have on their plates, and the bigger they make the portion the more they eat. Almost three decades ago the soda drink was 250 ml and it used to satisfy a person. However, now we have the one liter soda cup with a burger meal, and we think one liter is a normal size when ordering that particular meal.

Moreover, since we inherit our genes from our parents, and if our parents are overweight, most likely the children will also carry and pass on that gene (fat cells) to their children and the fat genes keep passing on to the following generations unless something changes along the way. Nevertheless, it doesn't mean we can't change, or if someone is overweight should use the parent's genes as an excuse.

Also, it doesn't mean our weight problems are not due to endocrine issues and hormone imbalances brought on to us by eating unhealthy foods full of xenoestrogens and toxins, taking medications we don't need, BPA products, stress, lack of sleep and exercise. All of us have responsibilities, which will be elaborated on later.

The social factor: the close social circle influences the risk of obesity. A New England Journal of Medicine published a research report in 2007, they tested a theory - your social circle influences factors such as physical activity and eating habits. For example, if your close social circle engages in physical activity or healthy eating, you're more likely to do so too.

The study followed more than 12,000 people over a period of 32 years and examined the influence of one person's weight gain among their social contacts. They found, having a close friend or spouse who became obese increases your chances of becoming obese by 37 and 57 percent, respectively.

These trends were not seen among neighbors, demonstrating that it's the habits of your close social circle which have the most influence on habits and may increase the risks of developing obesity.

Similarly, eating around others influences eating habits - people tend to eat more when around others and match their intake to that of their eating companions, according to a systematic review published in the American Journal of the Academy of Nutrition and Dietetics in 2014. Researchers aren't quite sure why this is so, but they theorize that people have a natural wish to conform to the standards of a group. The authors of the study point to this social influence on eating habits as a factor in weight gain and obesity. Based on their review of published data, they found that who you eat with influences what you choose to eat and how much you consume. This means, if you have friends you frequently eat with and who make poor food choices and eat large portion sizes, chances are you may be inclined to do the same.

Another factor associated with social influence and related to obesity is eating away from home play a major influence on weight-gain and obesity.

Whether you choose to eat with others or not, eating away from home is another habit that scientists warn may increase the risk of obesity. Researchers studied a Mediterranean population to evaluate the effects of eating away from home. For many years, citizens of Mediterranean countries ate most of their meals at home, until recent years. After evaluating the eating patterns of over 9,000 adults, researchers found that eating out was a significant risk factor for weight gain and obesity; people who ate out two or more times each week weighed more than those who ate at home. That is 855 participants became obese during the four-year follow-up.

Stress

Stress is one major factor in gaining weight and obesity. Stress changes our behavior, appetite and it stimulates what we're eating. Stress is also related to insulin resistance, metabolic syndrome and obesity in general.

The stress that is mentioned here is the same stress we have today in our society and life in general. It's the stress of paying the bills, losing a job, the mortgage, the credit card bills, health issues and the major one is the constant competitions which we face every day - whether at the job or simply "conformity" (keeping up with the joneses). The stresses are mentioned here could be basic to some people but those mentioned stresses are threatening - because under stress psychologically and biologically, we tend to reach for those easy foods to comfort us and calm us down, while holding on to those calories and to get ready for the next stress attack.

Since stress activates the same brain signals that famine and starvation do, this means the links between eating and stress are very similar. Stress makes people hungry simply by activating the same impulses that make them crave for high calories, and when we are stressed we tend to make less healthy choices because the brain is already overworking on getting rid of the present stress. Therefore, we go for the easier choices by choosing solid calories, high fat, high sweets and also high salty foods. Calories, fat, sugar and salt are what rewards the brain, especially a stressed brain. On a similar note, if you look around and observe, what kind of foods are the most available, cheapest to buy and easiest to reach? You'll only find "fast and junk foods". Therefore, when we're stressed we think of food and the first thing that comes to mind is fast and junk foods - because it's very rewarding to the brain (high fat, high sugar and high salt).

There is also another major threat that we all face when it comes to decision-making especially when we are under stress, which is "accepting suggestions". Often, we are very feeble, sensitive and receptive to suggestions when we are in a state of shock, stress and confusion. This is where marketing, advertisement and the media do their magic work. Therefore, stressed people start to buy and consume to feel at ease and feel happy again with what they buy and eat. It's sad when we started to seek comfort and happiness through products and things we buy, and start to love those things which don't love us back.

Hollywood

Note: *I will be releasing another book soon about hidden agendas and how this world is being run. Therefore, the following section will be further detailed in my new book.*

Since we only know what we know, most people don't know that there is a whole world hidden behind words, logos, emblems and symbols. In fact, the whole world is run by words, logos, emblems and symbols. The most efficient and effective way to run the world, control the masses, manipulate their thinking and direct their minds is by compensating those four in a form of entertainment "Hollywood".

The study of the world of the occult means simply to study the world of the hidden. Here's a brief occult history, the priesthood used to be called the Druids - who ruled ancient Europe. Those were ministers, priests, lawyers, nobles, politicians etc. The Druids held power within the society. Europe and their Anglo-American arm we now call the United States continue to be based on Druidic principles.

One of the most important symbols to the Druids was the magic wand made of the wood of the holly tree. Magicians, conductors and those in power all held magic wands or staffs. You were to play to their tune and dance to their beat, they directed you to play. The Hollywood of today is nothing other than a Druidic establishment. By the same token, Hollywood (magic wand = holly wood) is still being waved upon people to put them in a trance and direct their minds just as the Druids do.

Think about how Hollywood does what they do. A story is written which turns into a screen play, then actors are hired to act out the characters. Actors are paid to act out human emotions, the director is hired to direct the actors and place them exactly where he or she wants them within the shot. The director is responsible to the producer, who is responsible to the executive producer, who is ultimately producing the money for the film.

As the viewer you watch this story unfold on the big screen, the movie subliminally causes you to act in terms of what you just saw. Because of your emotional response to the film or show, you leave the theater or couch thinking this is how you normally act or react to certain situations, just the way the actor did in the movie.

That was only a brief explanation about how words could be hidden and masked, as well as symbols which are the language of the subconscious mind. The media does magic, and magic is simply words and symbols to manipulate the human's mind or control it. Moreover, there is another powerful and influential technique the media uses and that is "Propaganda".

Propaganda

Propaganda is what sells, whether it's a new food product, a new diet or a new medicine. A propaganda can also work perfectly for a new scientifically re-framed lie (in the name of science), a politically re-framed lie (in the name of the nation or national security), and the worst is religion (in the name of God). Any kind of propaganda is often delivered to the masses to sound more plausible and believable by a person of authority or simply can also be delivered by a paid scientist, news anchor, celebrity, politician or a religious figure depending on the type of the propaganda and the desired outcome of the lie.

Although a propaganda is not always negative, it's simply just a mode of communication used to manipulate or influence the opinion of groups to support a particular cause or belief. Over the centuries, propaganda has taken the form of artwork, films, speeches, and music, though it's not only limited to these forms of communication.

Moreover, propaganda very often involves a heavy emphasis on the benefits and virtues of one idea or group, while simultaneously distorting the truth or suppressing the counter-argument. For example, the Nazi party during World War II. Through speeches, posters, and films, the Nazis were able to convince the German people that the economic depression in the wake of World War I was not the result of governmental failure but was instead the fault of immigrants, communists, and other outsiders who were weakening the country. As they continued their rise to power, the Nazis frequently relied on propaganda to justify their actions and promote their beliefs. Another example, the Nazi party spread the message that Jews were responsible for the lack of jobs and were hoarding money; as a result, many Germans didn't object when Jewish people were imprisoned.

The Nazi party's actions might be the most commonly referenced and widely known example of propaganda, but the Nazis are only one of many groups who has used this technique. During World War II, the United States also frequently relied on propaganda for public support. Think of the image of Uncle Sam and the "I Want You" posters used to encourage people to join the military. Through heavy use, this image and slogan sent a message that joining the military was the patriotic and the right thing to do, particularly in the context of fighting evil.

Both of these examples demonstrate how propaganda is used to promote one idea while downplaying or ignoring the big picture. The Nazis used propaganda to deflect any personal responsibility for the economic depression and instead, pinned the blame on scapegoats (the Jewish people) whom Germans could direct their anger toward. The United States, on the other hand, celebrated joining the military as the patriotic thing to do, while ignoring the violent realities of war.

In recent times, the war on Iraq was also led by waves of propaganda supported by the United States and the coalitions. Many slogans were used such as the axis of evil, the weapon of mass destructions WMD, freeing the Iraqi people etc.

Similarly, the food industry also uses propaganda techniques, such as in chapter one where Earl Butz and the mass production of corn. As well as many campaigns were socially engineered by top propagandists such as Edward Bernays (the nephew of Sigmund Freud) and others who literally changed the 19th century.

Besides, since I'll be releasing another book further explaining such subjects, although it was important to briefly explain what propaganda is, so it helps to understand how the media and the corporations work.

Conformity

Conformity can be defined in psychology and sociology as a type of social influence involving a change in one's belief or to go along with the norms or a group of people - to be liked or accepted as an in-group, and also to avoid being the odd person, or the one who falls behind.

Conformity can also be used as a technique to control the masses, and the outcome can go to some extreme levels, such as Marxism, Nazism, Fascism and other extreme stages of conformity.

Additionally, there are several types of conformity. However here we are interested in the following few:

Normative Conformity, which involves changing one's behavior in order to fit in with the group. Internalization Conformity, which occurs when we change our behavior because we want to be like another person. And Informational Conformity is when conforming to a person or group of people who are in a position of being a source of information even in ambiguous situations.

Informational conformity can be dangerous in some cases because unfortunately experts or professionals are not always a reliable source of information since they also follow orders from a higher echelon. This leads us to the media, politicians, scientists, clergymen and other professionals which people conform to, and believe everything they say! For example, someone is in denial that plastic may cause cancer or fluoride in the water may cause neurological issues - simply because he/she saw a scientist on TV (who may have been paid by the same corporations that sell the fluoride or plastic or even associated with - to tell people it's safe). Also, that very scientist on TV maybe is not even a scientist or a doctor. He/she could be just a paid actor wearing a white gown and stethoscope, and reading a script written by a social engineer such as Edward Bernays who made people believe (till this very day) that bacon and eggs are a healthy breakfast!

This type of conformity is constantly occurring regularly. We're bombarded every moment with advertisements claiming safety and other false claims. Someone on TV wearing a chef's outfit and frying hamburgers and fries for a fast food junk restaurant advertisement, his outfit doesn't make him a chef cooking some fine food! A clown playing with children in an advertisement for fast, junk, high caloric and fat addictive foods doesn't mean he cares about your children! Someone is wearing a medical gown with a stethoscope around his neck on TV saying fluoride in the water is safe, that doesn't make the fluoride any safer! Informational conformity is the most effective and efficient tool for social engineers. Just remember that all wars are led by using false propaganda, and the same technique is still being used "informational conformity". They get a high ranked general (a war expert) or simply a serious looking paid actor wearing a uniform on TV saying we're facing a threat. Moments later, an advertisement to enroll in the "Corp", which stands for corporation if it's not already clear for some people. Later, you see a whole herd of patriots lining up to get enrolled believing they are doing the right thing. Those conformed people will even defend that false propaganda with everything they got even if knowing they are wrong. That is called "The Stockholm Syndrome". More about such cases will be in my next book.

The other two conformities which also play a major role in our health and diet are the normative conformity and internalization conformity. For example, there is an occasion such as a birthday where some unhealthy foods, drinks and desserts are served – and someone starts eating that unhealthy foods - knowing it's unhealthy. Such behavior simply occurs because everyone is eating and so the rest conform too. Most people tend to forget that a movie can be watched without a big bucket of popcorn full of fat butter, thousands of calories and 40 teaspoons of sugar family size soda drink. Also, a valentine can be celebrated without high caloric foods and chocolates full of fat. Moreover, we certainly can be blessed on Easter, Christmas, New Years and other religious/spiritual occasions without the high caloric, high carbohydrates, high fat, high salt and high sugar foods. God certainly won't be unpleased if such junk and unhealthy foods are not served and consumed on such occasions.

More will be explained about how we have started to mix food with our joy later in the following chapter. However, what you need to remember is to be independent in your thinking and decisions and be aware of yourself when you're conforming. The best way to achieve such awareness is to always think before you behave/act and always be cautious of what you buy and consume. Always think of the advertiser, not the advertisement and assess 'who is' and the 'why' behind this advertisement. Also, keep in mind, the more frequently you do something the more it will become normal to you. Brainwashing is nothing more than a repetitive pattern or message played or said over and over to you. Eventually, it will sink in deeply into your subconscious mind until it becomes part of your belief system.

Introduction - The Subconscious Mind

Note: *this introduction is based on Psychoanalysis, Neuro Linguistic Programming (NLP) and Hypnosis in relation to the subject. The purpose of this introduction is to give you a brief understanding of the mind and how it functions as to advertisements, subliminal suggestions and behavior. However, there is still a lot more about the subject - If you'd like to learn more about NLP and Hypnotherapy or if you wish to become a certified practitioner, more information can be found on The MindTech Institute website, www.TheMindTechInstitute.com*

The subconscious mind is a very powerful biological device, not only in terms of storing memories and information but also in having the ability to allow people to preform critical tasks unconsciously or when they are least conscious, as in "performing tasks on auto-pilot".

There are many mysteries about the subconscious mind. However, we know for sure that the major tasks of the subconscious mind are to store and retrieve information and the person to respond to the way they have been taught or programmed.

Many professionals in the field of psychology underestimate the capabilities of the subconscious mind, but make no mistake - the subconscious mind is even more powerful than most people think. It's true that the subconscious mind doesn't follow orders but there are ways to manipulate its patterns and to program, re-program and de-program it.

Through my experience and work in psychology and the numerous hypnosis hours that I've done with clients and students, I can confidently say that through hypnosis, (and I don't mean the hypnosis you get from the palm reading hypnosis corner shop), I mean the clinical supervised hypnosis, that it is one of the greatest natural tools to tap into the subconscious mind. It isn't a simple task as people may think, but it's certainly not complicated for those who are qualified hypnotherapists.

The subconscious mind is where every memory and thought have been stored since a person was born, in the mother's womb and some people believe even earlier. However, it is important to know that the subconscious mind stores memories and information throughout the whole person's life, as we store data on a hard drive. We can add more data, delete, program, edit, re-edit, manipulate and even add new ones without the awareness of the conscious mind. This technique is better known as subliminal and covert suggestions. Such work can be done without the person's awareness and this will cause the person to behave according to the new or the edited program. This will lead on to the next segment in this chapter and how that is being done on a regular basis, especially in the media and marketing!

Furthermore, the subconscious mind is one of three minds – as will follow, however, the three minds we have aren't three different brains! And in case if you're wondering about the difference between the brain and the mind - let's think of it this way; the brain is the physically visible organ and the mind is the invisible force such as thoughts. Yet everything the mind thinks or feels requires a physical response in the brain to be confirmed on the physical level as a physical experience, and then the experience will be stored as a filtered experience in the mind. Materialism has been debating the existence of the mind for a very long time, but what's the point of arguing its existence if its absence cannot be proven? We can't see the thought, but it doesn't mean the thought doesn't exist. We can't claim that the thought is a brain tissue which is made up of organic chemicals and fluids! It's a mistake to attribute a thought to physical things such as organs, cells, molecules, atoms etc.

Nonetheless, the three minds that are running the show are all connected and work with each other, sometimes directly and sometimes indirectly depending on the experience and event. They all fulfil a common purpose, which is to keep you alive, function well and safe. The failure of any of them will lead to imbalances in one's behavior, physiology and thinking.

The Subconscious Mind: is often referred to as the chief superior or the show runner. The subconscious mind is a great mystery, but no doubt it is where all information is stored and hidden for many generations. The subconscious mind doesn't think or make decisions, but there's certainly a very close coordination between the three minds especially the conscious and the subconscious. The subconscious mind is like a hard drive - everything you experienced, sensed, learnt and even thought is stored in it.

The subconscious mind is a permanent memory device, unlike the conscious mind. For example, it would be easy to remember your current cell phone number (conscious), but trying to remember your very first number would be difficult. However, the memory of your very first number isn't completely gone, in fact, it's stored in the subconscious. Additionally, there are techniques that can be used to retrieve information from the subconscious mind, even remembering experiences during the fetus state (mother's womb), through a hypnotic technique called "Regression".

Furthermore, throughout the years of my psychology studies and research regarding "Past Life Experience", we have found some very significant breakthroughs in such phenomena. It may not be as what some beliefs claim, but certainly, there is some truth to it, and it can be explained scientifically.

Another important thing worth mentioning in regards to the subconscious mind is "self-preservation". The subconscious mind is very protective over the person him/herself; it might put a person in a coma just to save his/her life, especially in severe pain cases. The subconscious mind can also turn an abused fit person to become obese - in order to become unattractive to their abusers and to cease the abusing act. The subconscious will do anything to save the person's life, even if it's going to cause the person illnesses and other problems. In many cases, the subconscious mind may also create amnesia (forgetting an experience) of a traumatic event in order to get the person to move on in life. That's a part of self-preservation.

The Conscious Mind is the thinker and decision maker. It is rational, analytical, has very short term memory and keeps you safe by risk assessing situations and events. The conscious mind essentially identifies incoming information. This information received through any of the six senses: visual, sound, smell, taste, touch, or feeling. Your conscious mind is continually observing and categorizing what is going on around you.

For example, if you were to jump from a certain distance, your conscious mind will analyze and rationalize the safety of your jump and decide if you should jump or not from such distance to avoid getting injured.

Also, short-term memories and will-power are a part of the conscious mind. As a result, many people fail to quit smoking, stop drinking, quit drugs or a certain food – because often they create lots of hypes but no actions will be taken. The reason is because usually, habits and addictions including eating, smoking, drinking, drugs etc. are in the subconscious mind. Consequently, when most people try to quit or stop a habit, they get back to it after a while because they used "will-power" when they tried to quit and will power is in the conscious mind. Will-power runs on adrenalin, and adrenalin has a certain time to drop again to its natural level. Hence, the hype will fade away. Furthermore, since the conscious mind has short term memory, so as will-power. It's a short time hype and then will fade out, and later it will be forgotten. That is the reason why most people fail to quit something because they were working on consciously rather than subconsciously where it is stored in the first place. Thus, a habit must be edited, reprogrammed or deprogrammed from the subconscious mind by using some powerful techniques such as hypnosis to get into the subconscious.

The Unconscious Mind: The unconscious mind often does essential things such as the Immune system, respiratory system, heartbeat, eyes blinking and other automatic bodily functions.

The subconscious mind and accepting suggestions

One of the most powerful mind control and brainwashing technique is "repetition". If you say a lie over and over again no matter how ridiculous the lie may sound, people will eventually believe it. Whenever anything is repeated times after times people will eventually accept it, believe it and later defend it.

Another good example is when a new song comes out - regardless how ridiculous the song might be, all radio stations and media outlets start to play it - multiple or several times every day, and then you find yourself singing that same ridiculous song! That is because the song was repeated much time in the same day by many sources. The mind will eventually conform to the repetitions regardless what and how it is. The same instance goes with a burger, medicine, product and even presidential elections. The more the word, song, news, or story is repeated, the more people will begin to believe it and defend it even if it's a lie.

World class propagandist Joseph Goebbels (1897 – 1945) was Adolf Hitler's propaganda minister in Nazi Germany. Joseph Goebbels said, "If you tell a lie big enough and keep repeating it, people will eventually come to believe it." He also said, "The most brilliant propagandist technique will yield no success unless one fundamental principle is borne in mind constantly - it must confine itself to a few points and repeat them over and over".

The most effective and efficient time for the mind to be manipulated is when people are in a state of fear, shock, confusion and depression. Such technique works effectively well especially when the programming (accepting suggestions) is delivered by an authority figure such as a president, minister, military commander, doctor, engineer, manager, religious leader, clergyman, news reporter, celebrity, teachers, parents or someone with a high regarded position or status in society, group or even for an individual - and that is "Informational Conformity"!

Additionally, for any suggestion to be promptly accepted by the subconscious mind, it must be delivered in a positive form. Therefore, most negative suggestions wear a positive mask to trick the subconscious mind. That technique is called "reframing or spin". Another process is being used along with reframing is called "back masking and subliminal messaging", many of which can be found in TV advertisements and songs.

Subliminal advertisements

There have been numerous cases where subliminal techniques been used in advertising and for propaganda and advertisement purposes

A subliminal message is a signal or message designed to bypass the "critical factor of the subconscious mind" or more commonly known as the guard of the subconscious mind. Its purpose is to pass below the normal limits of perception. For example, it might be inaudible to the conscious mind (but audible to the subconscious mind) or might be an image transmitted briefly and unperceived consciously and yet perceived subconsciously.

Subliminal perception or cognition is a subset of unconscious cognition where the forms of unconscious cognition also include attending to one signal in a noisy environment while unconsciously keeping track of other signals (e.g. one voice out of many in a crowded room) and tasks done automatically (e.g. driving a car).

Let's think of it this way, subliminal messages in advertisements are sensory related stimuli are aimed below a person's level of conscious perception, or too fast to be detected by the conscious mind. The two most common types are visual stimuli and audio stimuli. Visual-based subliminal messages such as quickly flashed images before the brain has time to process them. Audio subliminal stimuli may be played below the audible volume, or similarly masked by other sounds and noises, or recorded backwards in a process called "back-masking". It might be too fast for the conscious mind's filters to detect them and categorize them, but as everything else is experienced or collected by any of our senses will be stored in the subconscious mind. Then, the effect of such messages take their course of action whenever you hear that tone, see the symbol or logo again. Also, you will even fall into the emotional state which the advertisement has anchored you on, and you will respond accordingly. This process is called "activating the triggers" or "firing (activating) the anchors".

The subconscious mind often relates everything to symbols (visual), tones (auditory) and emotional events (kinesthetic). The suggestions will be more effective when it's compounded by all our major senses, such as our visual, auditory, kinesthetic, olfactory (smelling) and gustatory (tasting) senses - and that's what we see in most advertisements.

How do subliminal messages and advertisements work?

All is needed for a message to be subliminally implanted in a person's mind is to bypass the critical factor of the subconscious mind. That is the guard assigned to protect the subconscious mind from unfiltered and categorized information – which is a process analyzed by the conscious mind. The filters will categorize the event or experience (seeing, tasting, smelling, felling, hearing etc.), label the event or experience in whichever department they belong to, and then store them.

The process of bypassing the critical factor of the subconscious mind can be achieved in many ways. However, since it's a process of study and it takes some series of lessons during our Hypnosis Training at The MindTech Institute. Here is a brief explanation of how it works only in the media, which will help you to understand the following segment.

Bypassing the critical factor of the subconscious mind in a visual advertisement - involves confusing the conscious mind with rapid flickers or flashes during the advertisement (most of those flickers and flashes aren't detectable by the conscious mind because they are faster than what the conscious mind can perceive, but you can easily see them by filming the TV screen through a video camera). While the flickers and flashes are running, a frame which contains the subliminal message is already inserted within the running frames will pass while you're watching (without you're noticing) and will be stored in your subconscious usually with a program (which is the content of the message).

For example, industry standard motion picture film traditionally is filmed at 24 frames per second (some new movies are being filmed at 48 fps). Nevertheless, one frame contains the subliminal message will be inserted within the 24 frames. The message may contain a logo, slogan, image, message or any suggestion such as "buy it now, you love it etc."

At this stage, the subconscious mind had detected an uncategorized frame, but it may pass through because the person is in a trance caused by the light, flickers music etc. - and also because the message is being masked by a positive frame. This confusion will make the person more receptive, especially because the person is already in a trance of (watching the TV). Consequently, all these flashing flickers are numbing the brain with waves and images, it's almost impossible for the conscious mind to keep up with such speed to do its job (filtering and categorizing), especially if there is music or voices involved. Eventually, the information will be stored and anchored successfully in the subconscious mind.

When the information (message) is stored in the subconscious mind, it can be easily triggered by activating the anchors which have been created during the advertisement resulting in making you like the product and make you believe that you need it. The trigger is activated every time you see the logo or hear the tune of the advert etc.

An advert example, you see an advertisement of a burger on TV, they anchor you with the messages when you watch it over and over. Then, you go for a drive and you see the logo of that junk burger. The visual anchor (trigger) is already being activated (when you saw the logo) - then all of a sudden you feel hungry - and you start getting the urge to pull over to satisfy that urge by eating the junk food meal. The fact is you didn't need the burger nor you were hungry in the first place, that was the power of that anchor led you to think you were hungry. Moreover, this behavior can become an addiction designed to make you subconsciously accept it - and making you believe that you're enjoying it even if it tastes like dirt. The program in your mind is already being installed as "it's delicious", and that's why you think it tastes good. You may also defend that junk unhealthy food if someone told you it doesn't taste good, even though you're not being paid by the junk company to defend them! You're actually paying them for that piece of junk which is causing you all kinds of health issues. And as you already know by now, once you defend something and knowing its dangers to you and onto others, you have then got the "Stockholm Syndrome" (loving and defending your abusers), essentially and purely caused by brainwashing you and the masses through marketing and addictive substances.

Furthermore, usually children are more receptive than adults, and that's why they get excited every time you pass next to the famous burger junk food store.

Lastly, I'll share with you a story of how the mind can be easily manipulated. In my early study years, I used to do stage hypnosis shows, and during the shows, I used to pick some people from the audience to come up on the stage. I used to put the person in a trance (light hypnotic state, similar to when you're watching the TV) and then put suggestions in the person's head. I would tell the person something untrue that would become his/her reality. I would place an onion in a person's hand with a per-suggestion that it's an apple (as I programmed the person to believe that the onion is an apple, similarly as the advertisement programs you as this burger is so delicious). I used to tell the person to eat the onion, and would completely believe it is an apple. The person would look at it and swear it's an apple and tastes like an apple, (it's the same when you eat that burger you may swear it tastes good, even if it tastes like dirt). This is a very simple and basic reprogramming mind patterns which we teach to hypnotists Practitioner Level. Then, you can imagine what a hypnotist Master Practitioner can do!

If I, one man on a stage, or our hypnosis "practitioner level" students can reprogram someone's mind in such a way, then what do you think the whole media empire can do? They can absolutely change history at any given time and people will believe it.

Nonetheless, subliminal messaging and covert hypnotic suggestions aren't all bad and evil. Otherwise, I won't be teaching hypnosis, Neuro Linguistic Programming (NLP) to Practitioner and Master Practitioner Levels for the obvious ethical reasons. Such techniques are like a language, can be used in a positive or in a negative way, or for a good reason or as for destroying others. Many people can use these techniques in therapy and education, and we have achieved some amazing results for those who are in need of such help. For example, how wonderful it is when you can re-program yourself or someone who is addicted to smoking, chocolate, sugar, drugs etc. and to give up all these addictions. Also, how amazing it is when you re-program yourself to become more successful and achieve the results you want in your life. That's not bad at all! However, it is bad when Monsanto replaces a healthy organic food with GMO and tell us it's good and safe. Or when the media pull out some propaganda on us - by masking the truth with falsehood to convince us that there's a boogeyman hiding in a cave, and we have to go to war to kill millions of innocents all based on lies and other mind manipulation effects to serve their agendas. This is how things work in the media world. And knowledge is the best way to protect yourself and others.

Unfortunately, the world is not run by good capable people. The world is run by people who are capable of many things but good doesn't seem to be one of them.

As George Carlin said, "It's a big club and you ain't in it. You and I are not in the big club. By the way, it's the same big club they use to beat you over the head with all day long when they tell you what to believe. All day long beating you over the head with their media telling you what to believe, what to think and what to buy. The table has tilted folks. The game is rigged and nobody seems to notice. Nobody seems to care… because the owners of this country know the truth. It's called the American Dream because you have to be asleep to believe it . . ."

"If you're not careful, the newspapers will have you hating the people who are being oppressed, and loving the people who are doing the oppressing."

- Malcolm X

"It's easier to fool people than to convince them they have been fooled."

- Mark Twain

"Democracy is a con game. It's a word invented to placate people to make them accept a given institution. All institutions sing, 'We are free.' The minute you hear 'freedom' and 'democracy', watch out… because in a truly free nation, no one has to tell you you're free."

- Jacque Fresco

Suggestions

Desiderius Erasmus wrote, "Prevention is better than cure". And similarly, Benjamin Franklin also wrote, "An ounce of prevention is worth a pound of cure". In addition, the purpose of this segment is to focus on preventions. Although, it is very hopeful to think that there's a universal solution, but I'd rather keep logical at this stage because of the way the world is running and the powerful people who are running the show.

Needless to say, prevention doesn't need any approval but from oneself. We don't need to wait for the world to change for the better, but we can all start with ourselves and in our own homes. Furthermore, the following suggestions are encouraged to be considered and consulting your physician or doctor is highly recommended.

Facts about Fluoride You Need to Know

Many people assume, if the government allows fluoride in the water, it must be safe – but it's not. Nevertheless, it would be very hard to believe that the government is so concerned about your teeth while all these toxic and poisonous substances in food products which you have read about so far are flooding the markets. If it's as safe as they claim, then why can't you just go and get fluoride tablets without prescription from your doctor?

What is fluoride? It depends on who you ask – and you will defiantly get different "spin" answers from dentists and health bureaucrats. For example, dentists will tell you, fluoride is natural and exists naturally in virtually all water supplies and even in various brands of bottled water. They will also tell you fluoride is good, reduces tooth decay and safe if it's used between 0.0 - 0.7 parts per million. However, unfortunately, many dentists aren't researches and they just repeat what they have learnt to say without a close investigating the matter. Let's first clear up the natural claim of fluoride - fluoridation advocates often use this spin "it's natural" to support its safety, however naturally occurring substances are not automatically safe to us (think of arsenic, for instance).

Furthermore, according to the Review of Toxicological Literature, the National Institute of Environmental Health Sciences, the fluoride added to most water supplies is not the naturally occurring fluoride [which many dentists think it is] but rather a poison called fluorosilicic acid, which is a toxic waste from the production of fertilizer. Or simply as they call them "wet scrubbers" – which are pollution control devices used by the phosphate industry such as; those generated by aluminum, steel, fertilizer factories, coal burning power plants and in the production of glass and cement, gaseous fluoride and other process waste byproducts and others - to capture fluoride gases produced in the production of commercial fertilizer. In the past, when the industry let these gases escape, vegetation became scorched, crops destroyed, and cattle crippled. Today, with our sophisticated air-pollution control technology, less of the fluoride escapes into the atmosphere. However, the impacts of the industry's fluoride emissions are still being felt, although more subtly, by millions of people – people who, for the most part, do not live anywhere near a phosphate plant. That's because, after being captured in the scrubbers, the fluoride acid (hydrofluorosilicic acid), a classified hazardous waste, is barreled up and sold, unrefined, to communities across the country. Communities add hydrofluorosilicic acid to their water supplies as the primary fluoride chemical for water fluoridation. Even if you don't live in a community where fluoride is added to water, you'll still be getting a dose of it through cereal, soda, juice, beer, many bottled water, vegetables, processed meats and any other processed foods and drinks manufactured with fluoridated water. Moreover, these industries would have to pay dearly to dispose of their fluoride if they could not sell it to municipalities for adding to their tap water. "In other words," says William Hirzy, a Senior EPA scientist, "fluoride that otherwise would be an air and water pollutant is no longer a pollutant as long as it's poured into your reservoir. The solution to pollution is dilution and in this case, the dilution is your drinking water."

Here is a common sense question, since the whole revenue of dentists is heavily relying on bad teeth and cleaning teeth – so, why would those dentists who are advocates for such toxic to insist so passionately on keeping the water fluoridated?! The answer is simple, it has nothing to do with the health of your teeth but with what they are trained to say. Also, why governments insist on fluoridating water supposedly "for the health of our teeth" while most of those governments don't even pay your dental bill?! The dental bills are paid by the individual and not as "bulk-billing" or Medicare [which is Australia's health care system that covers health care costs, similarly like Medicaid in the U.S.] As a matter of fact, ingesting fluoride – which is a sickening cocktail of arsening, barium, beryllium, cadmium, copper, lead, mercury and other deadly toxins isn't worth the health risks to be even considered to save our teeth!

On the contrary, fluoride is bad for the teeth. In 2007 the American Dental Association (ADA) first warned that parents of infants younger than a year old "should consider using water that has no or low levels of fluoride" when mixing baby formula, due to concerns about fluorosis. Exposure to high levels of fluoride results in a condition known as fluorosis, in which tooth enamel becomes discolored. The condition can eventually lead to badly damaged teeth.

Also, in 2010, the Journal of the American Dental Association published a study that once again found, contrary to what most people have been told: fluoride is actually bad for your teeth. The study showed increased fluorosis risk among infants who were fed infant formula reconstituted with fluoride-containing water, as well as for those using fluoridated toothpaste. The authors noted: "Results suggest that prevalence of mild dental fluorosis could be reduced by avoiding ingestion of large quantities of fluoride from reconstituted powdered concentrate infant formula and fluoridated dentifrice".

Dental fluorosis is not the only risk from early ingestion of fluoride. Fluoride exposure can also negatively impact brain development, resulting in both learning and behavioral disorders.

It is often claimed that fluoridated water is the main reason the United States has had a large decline in tooth decay over the past 60 years. This same decline in tooth decay, however, has occurred in all developed countries, most of which have never added any fluoride to their water. Today, according to data from the World Health Organization, there is no discernible difference in tooth decay between the minority of developed countries that fluoridate water and the majority that do not.

Fluoridation advocates have long claimed that the safety of fluoridation is beyond scientific debate. However, according to the well-known toxicologist, Dr. John Doull, who chaired the National Academy of Science's review on fluoride, the safety of fluoridation remains "unsettled" and "we have much less information than we should, considering how long it has been going on." In 2006, Doull's committee at the NAS published an exhaustive 500-page review of fluoride's toxicity. The report concludes that fluoride is an "endocrine disruptor" and can affect many things in the body, including the bones, the brain, the thyroid gland, the pineal gland, and even blood sugar levels.

Far from giving fluoride a clean bill of health, the NAS called upon scientists to investigate if current fluoride exposures in the United States are contributing to chronic health problems, like bone disorders, thyroid disease, low intelligence [low IQ], dementia, obesity and diabetes, particularly in people who are most vulnerable to fluoride's effects. These recommendations highlight that—despite 60 years of fluoridation—many of the basic studies necessary for determining the program's safety have yet to be conducted.

Water fluoridation first began back in the 1940s, the medical profession believed fluoride needed to be ingested to be most effective in preventing cavities. This was why fluoride was added to water and pills—because these are things that people swallow.

However, nowadays it is now widely recognized that fluoride's main benefit does not actually come from ingestion, it comes from fluoride's topical contact with teeth - a fact that even the CDC has now acknowledged in (1999) - Morbidity and Mortality Weekly Report 48: 933-40.

Despite all the risks and health issues of fluoride, this might be shocking to some people but fluoride supplements have never been actually approved by the FDA. Fluoride "supplements" are designed to provide children with the same dose of fluoride they would receive by drinking fluoridated water. Unlike other dietary supplements! You can't just walk into a grocery store and buy a fluoride supplement. Because of fluoride's toxicity, you can only buy a fluoride "supplement" if you have a doctor's prescription. Yet, although federal law requires that prescription drugs be approved as safe and effective by the FDA – however, the FDA has never approved fluoride supplements for the prevention of tooth decay [you can check the FDA's letters confirming this fact, see: www.fluoridealert.org/researchers/FDA/not-approved/]. In fact, the only fluoride supplements the FDA has reviewed, have been rejected. So, with fluoridation, that is added to the water is a prescription-strength dose of a drug that has never been approved by the FDA. In other words, it's forced medication for the masses and there are more than thousand doctors, professors and professionals around the world who condemn this forced neurotoxic - endocrine - disrupting drug on the masses especially without the public consent. The basics of medical ethics are "a doctor/s can NOT give a drug to the patient without the patient's consent" and fluoride is "a drug" has been given to the masses [not patients] without their consent. This is a total violation of one's right and clearly exercised as it's commonly known in political science as "an Orwellian State Law".

The health risks of fluoride are far worse than a tooth cavity. And just to be fair and not to point all fingers at your state government, the real corporate in this matter is the bureaucrats who are spinning the information before it gets to the decision makers in some governments. The unfortunate thing is, we usually expect politicians to spin but we shouldn't expect civil servants such as dentists and some medical doctors to spin.

Suggestions; there is many doctors, dentists and other professionals advice to avoid the exposure to fluoride. And if you're drinking water is fluoridated, you can get any reverse osmosis filter at a very considerable price as long as it is for fluoride. If you have children: offer a healthy organic diet combined with teaching good dental hygiene habits as an alternative to fluoride dental products and supplements.

Alkaline VS Acidic Diet

The human body is equipped with very sensitive internal balance mechanism between Alkaline and Acid. When the balance is more toward Alkaline the body will be overflowing with energy and heavily armed with its immune system. The body will also rapidly disposes of fat. And the skin, bones, tissues and cells will regenerate faster keeping the body young and rejuvenated. But there is a problem, most of us in the western world are too "Acidic". And sadly our western diet has been exported to other countries around the world in the past few decades, leading most of the world to become also too acidic.

Too acidic means you'll gain and hold on fat, attract diseases and viruses, age quicker than you should, have a lack of energy and other issues. The reason we are too acidic is because our lifestyle consists of pesticides, alcohol, tobacco, fast and junk food, stress, radiation, chemicals, pharmaceutical drugs, soft drinks, excessive caffeine, energy drinks, artificial sweeteners, fluoride in water, fried foods, processed foods, sugar, un-natural juice, imitation foods, air pollutions etc. all the above cause acid in your body. Although, our bodies are in a constant fight to keep us balanced as in the alkaline zone, but the mission gets harder with what our lifestyle and food consists nowadays.

According to Dr. Melinda Ratini, A pH level measures how acid or alkaline something is. A pH of 0 is totally acidic, while a pH of 14 is completely alkaline. A pH of 7 is neutral. Those levels vary throughout your body. Your blood is slightly alkaline, with a pH between 7.35 and 7.45. Your stomach is very acidic, with a pH of 3.5 or below, so it can break down foods. And your urine changes, depending on what you eat -- that's how your body keeps the level in your blood steady.

Furthermore, pH stands for the power of hydrogen, which is a measurement of the hydrogen ion concentration in the body. The pH of 7 is considered to be neutral. A pH less than 7 is said to be acidic and solutions with a pH greater than 7 are basic or alkaline. Our ideal pH is slightly alkaline - 7.30 to 7.45. You can test your pH levels regularly by using a piece of litmus paper in your saliva or urine first thing in the morning before eating or drinking anything.

Below is the pH scale:

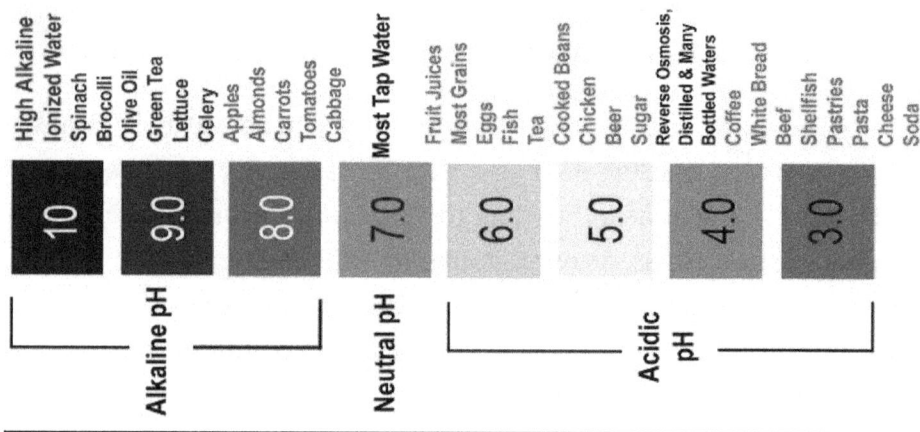

High Alkaline / Ionized Water	Spinach / Brocolli / Olive Oil / Green Tea	Lettuce / Celery / Apples / Almonds / Carrots / Tomatoes / Cabbage	Most Tap Water	Fruit Juices / Most Grains / Eggs / Fish / Tea	Cooked Beans / Chicken / Beer / Sugar	Reverse Osmosis, Distilled & Many Bottled Waters / Coffee / White Bread	Beef / Shellfish / Pastries / Pasta / Cheese / Soda
10	9.0	8.0	7.0	6.0	5.0	4.0	3.0

Alkaline pH | Neutral pH | Acidic pH

Quick facts:

It takes around 33 glasses of water to naturalize one glass of cola or soda drink! When your body is too acidic, your body will try everything to get more Alkaline. Seemingly it sounds good but actually, this is when the trouble starts as I'll explain to you the good and the bad sides as follow:

The good side; your body stores some acid in your fat to prevent it from harming. But the bad side is, your body then holds onto the fat for protection. That's the weight loss struggle (getting rid of weight struggle).

Another good side, your body will balance out alkaline levels in your body if you're more acidic than alkaline - your body will find alkaline from elsewhere in your body, such as your bones and teeth. But the downside is, your bones and teeth get their life drained out of them and they become frail and decay. That's the arthritis battle and that's why people shrink as they age.

The good side, the acid settles away from healthier organs. The bad side is, instead it hits your weakest organs that are already prone to diseases or hereditary cancer. That means cancer cells become dormant if you are of pH 7.4.

The major and worst one of all that it contaminates your blood! Think of it this way, your body is like a vehicle and when you run it on dirty oil you will have all kinds of issues such as; causing the engine parts to wear and tear quickly, not operating as it was designed to, become unreliable and lose its power etc. Engine oil is to vehicles as blood is to humans but your body is more vital. Your red blood cells deliver oxygen to the tissues, collect carbon dioxide and convey vitamins and sugars as well as amino acids. Each red blood cell is surrounded by a negative charge in order to bounce off each other and delivering their work efficiently. However, when you're too acidic your red blood cells lose their negative charge and they start to stick together, they sludge through the body at slow speed struggling to absorb water, nutrients, oxygen and can't expel unhealthy toxins. And that will lead to poisoning, and you'll feel a loss of energy even if you're getting enough sleep! It's the same thing the blood does after a person drinks alcohol. It is very possible for a person to get alkalized nowadays simply by choosing more alkaline foods and drinks as recommended by most medical doctors.

You may ask and consult your physician for more information about what is best for you.

Cancer – Conventional Vs Alternative Cancer Treatments

"More than 40 years after Nixon launched the war on cancer, we are not much closer to curing the disease. Why? Because finding a cure is the wrong goal." - Dr. Margaret Cuomo.

In his 1971 State of the Union address, President Richard M. Nixon promised Americans that he would begin "an extensive campaign to find a cure for cancer." He said, "The time has come to America to launch an extensive campaign to find a cure for cancer."

More than 40 years later, President Barack Obama similarly said, "Our recovery plan will invest in electronic health records, a new technology that will reduce errors, bring down costs, ensure privacy, and save lives. It will launch a new effort to conquer a disease that has touched the life of nearly every American including me by seeking a cure for cancer in our time."

Since the war on cancer began on 1971, more than 14,800,000 Americans have died in some form of the disease. 1500 die every day. And 565,000 death of men, women and children in 2009 alone! Charles B. Simone, M.MS., M.D, said in an interview, "from 1920 to the present time we had made little to no progress in the treatment of adult cancers. So, a person who gets prostate cancer or breast cancer today will live as long as a person who got it in 1920. No big change. So, all the radiation therapies that we began in the 10s and 20s, combinations of chemotherapies in the 60s, immunotherapies that we began in the 70s, CAT scans, MRI scans you name it, billions of billions of research dollars that we have thrown into this whole area of cancer research and treatment, little or no significant progress in the treatments of adults cancers".

So, technically what they do with cancer, they will burn it, cut it out or try to poison it and in the process will be poisoning the whole person's body along with cancer, and that will lead to further treatments and further treatment is more money for the cancer industry. The cancer business is worth an estimated 1 trillion dollars industry, they are not just going to pack up and go away. Think about it, only in America there is more than 1 million Americans are diagnosed with cancer every year. It's estimated, a cancer treatment will cost around 50000 dollars, and that will make 50 billion dollars a year to this industry only from America alone. All these people will found themselves in a tunnel that will change their lives for many years. And will be caught up with apparently an endless chain of medical tests, examinations, second opinions, medications, new tests, surgical operations, support therapies and follow-up checks. They will find themselves at the complete mercy of the disease. While in that tunnel, each patient feeds an enormous medical system that employs hundreds of thousands of people and generates billions of dollars for the medical and pharmaceutical industry – from research laboratories to medical schools, and from prevention clinics to worldwide drug sales. Today this cancer medical system is massive and very expensive - and it needs its patients in order to survive. Therefore, they will not work on a cure to find an end to the disease, but they will keep working on finding more treatments for the disease.

Moreover, there are a lot of alternative cancer treatments which are proven to successfully cure cancers. Those alternative cancer treatments have been tried and proven by people who were diagnosed with cancer and did not go through the conventional treatments. Those people survived and are a living proof. You can find tones of legit stories of cancer survivals without going through chemotherapies and other radiation conventional treatments. However, why you will never hear about those alternative treatments? Why have people to go overseas to seek alternative treatments? Why don't most doctors know about these alternative treatments? Even if doctors knew about such alternative treatments they will not tell you. Simply because they will lose their medical license and other harsh consequences will follow including imprisonment and in some cases even lose their lives! I urge you to look up Dr. Sebi who cured cancers, AIDS, diabetes and many other diseases. Dr. Sebi was arrested in Honduras and mysteriously died in prison on August 6, 2016. He was certainly one of many who faced similar consequence.

If conventional therapies have such limited results, then why the medical profession isn't willing to investigate alternative approaches? The answer to this question can be simply found in some historic events that took place almost a century ago when official medicine finally manage to gain the upper hand on the so-called empirical doctors who cured patients with herbs and natural remedies. In the 1800s, people had a choice to use either doctor called "allopath" or natural healers called "empirics or homeopath". The two groups waged a bitter philosophical debates. The allopathic doctors called their approach "heroic medicine" — they believed the physician must aggressively drive the disease from the body. The allopath used three main techniques, they bled the body to drain out the bad humors, they gave huge doses of toxic minerals such as mercury and led to displace the original disease, and they used surgeries but it was a brutal procedure before anesthesia and infection control. Few patients were willing to have surgeries, while most patients feared allopathic methods all together. It was widely known that with allopathic treatments the patients died of the cure.

The drug industry grew out of the booming patent medicine business and the doctors changed educational standards and licensing regulations to exclude the empiricists (homeopathic doctors) by forming the American Medical Associations (AMA). Soon later, only AMA approved doctors could legally practice medicine. In a brief of 20 years, the AMA came to dominate the medical practice. Also, organized medicine launched an immediate propaganda campaign to associates the empiricists (homeopathic doctors) with "Quacks" and the code name for the competition was "Quackery".

And now, here's the shocking part which most people don't know, modern medical doctors get only 10 hours of nutritional training in their whole medical degree! Also, most of the nutritional information they receive during their 10 hours of training are mostly inaccurate or outdated. In other words, they are just trained to prescribe drugs. The average wife of those physicians knows more about nutrition than he does, but they sure they know their drugs very well. If you go to your typical doctor today regardless what he/she is, the chances are you're going to walk out of there with a prescription. Why? Because that's what he/she has been trained to do.

Furthermore in finding who the real "Quacks" are, the companies that make up the pharmaceutical industry among the largest corporations in the world. Together, all these businesses came to be known as "Big Pharma". According to Drug Watch, in 2014, their combined sales was over $1 trillion with Johnson & Johnson, Pfizer, Abbot Laboratories, Merck and Eli Lilly leading the pack. In the U.S, the main source of Big Pharma's enormous profits is from sales prescription medication, and since these drugs can only be prescribed by medical professionals or better say AMA approved doctors, most of the industry promotional and marketing activities are directed to doctors, pharmacists and other healthcare providers.

Larry D. Sasich, PharmD, MPH, FASHP, of Public Citizen's Health Research Group, explained, "This starts out in the first year of medical school, and any many medical schools even the incoming students that are two years away from seeing a patient will start getting gifts from the pharmaceutical industry. And as the student gets further along in their medical education, the iterations and the gifts escalate to lunches, to dinners."

Also, Gene Carbona (Former Pharmaceutical Industry Insider and Current Executive Director of Sales, The Medical Letter) stated, "No matter where you spend money, in pharmaceutical promotion – whether it's in sample distribution, educational programming, non-educational programming, champagne brunches, happy hours, NY Jets tickets - no matter where you spend the money, you make money. And my boss always told me, there will always be more funding, spend what you can. In fact, if I give you $100,000 to spend, Gene, I want you to spend $200,000." So, now you know who the real "Quacks" are and you know what really works!

Awareness

The whole world must understand by now that the answer is not another pill, but it's about eating healthy, lifestyle and awareness. Awareness is one of the major preventions in regards to health and a healthy lifestyle.

It's the awareness of what you're feeding yourself, and most importantly is when you should eat. If you're aware of when you're hungry, then you're certainly aware of when you're not! This is a simple and basic test you can do before you eat. When you feel hungry and decide to go to eat, ask yourself - do I feel like eating an apple? If your answer is yes, it means you're hungry (because a hungry person will eat anything). If you say no, it means you're just bored or maybe have the association of joy and food syndrome. Therefore, awareness is very important and needed, as well as to be consciously aware of your actions by building that self-awareness with knowledge.

Losing weight Vs getting rid of weight

The "Yo-Yo Diet" usually happens when someone tries to slim down or get fitter. The Yo-Yo diet was first explained by Prof. Kelly D. Brownell and colleagues. The definition of the Yo-Yo diet is when people try to lose weight, and then they regain the same weight back which they have worked hard to get rid of. The Yo-Yo Diet is caused by many factors, and a major one is psychological rather than physical.

One of the major psychological factors of the Yo-Yo diet is because the subconscious mind takes everything literally and seriously based on its nature, and generally because the subconscious mind doesn't think or analyze as the conscious mind does. Therefore, the subconscious mind only does things as in "by commands"! Think of it this way, the subconscious mind is like the Aladdin's lamp, or better known as the genie in the bottle. The genie's job is only to preform and manifest your commands, not to think of what you command him! So, whether you say "I want lots of money" or "I want to be poor", the genie will grant you your commands without thinking of what your commands are. Similarly, the subconscious mind doesn't think but, it only acts. That's why you must be careful of what you say to yourself. If you say I'm ugly or fat, the subconscious mind will act as "your wish (suggestion) is my command" and you'll become as you suggested. Therefore, you better speak highly of yourself - to yourself, or don't say anything if you have nothing positive to say to yourself.

Back to the Yo-Yo Diet, when people say I want to lose 30 pounds of weight; they may lose that weight, but soon after might re-gain it all back - because the suggestion (command) used was to "lose". In the same respect, what do you do when you lose something?! You look everywhere for it to find it and to put it back where it was. The same thing goes with the subconscious mind. You lost 30 pounds, your subconscious mind will look everywhere for it, find it and to put it back on because it is the subconscious mind's job to protect you and what belongs to you. You may be thinking "but the subconscious mind should know that extra weight is making me sick"! Well, no! Because its job is not to think, and it doesn't think or calculate, it's just a memory storing department and a very powerful influence on your being.

Therefore, in order to avoid such suggestion, you better say, "I will get rid of the excess or unnecessary weight." That's much safer to say, and a SMART goal plan is to specify how much weight you want to get rid of. Also, the subconscious mind doesn't like the word "diet" because it has the word "die" in it! You can use words such as "eating healthier or eating smarter, eating better etc." If you remember from the previous chapter "the subconscious mind doesn't take negative suggestions", and the word "die" most likely is negative to the majority of people. This is a reason why people will drift away from a diet every time they say or hear the word "diet" because the subconscious mind will do the opposite of a negative suggestion!

Awareness also plays a major role here, you need self-awareness in order to start treating yourself with a higher regards because you know your subconscious mind is recording everything you're saying and thinking about yourself and others. Everything will be taken literally and acted upon accordingly. So, think it right, say it right and do it right!

The Food Emotional Note

Many people act when they eat as they are on some auto-pilot mode. They don't think about what they are eating and the kind of foods they are combining, the portion they are eating, and certainly forget how much they eat. When people are in that mode, it means they are in the trance of eating, and totally on auto-pilot mode (subconscious mode). As you already know by now, "habits" exist in the subconscious mind, and you know that eating on such mode becomes a habit. Therefore, it's recommended for the auto-pilot mode eaters to put some conscious activity (conscious mind as in analytical and rational) during eating to reduce the auto-pilot mode eating (subconscious) habit. On the contrary, when there is conscious activity in a behavior or state, the subconscious will not be involved or engaged in that behavior or state, as in direct engagement!

The best solution is to be more conscious of what you're eating. Write down what you ate and the portions. Also, write down the feelings and taste involved in each food. This technique will increase your conscious activity and give you an analytical and rational decision of what/when/how much you're eating, and also will increase your self-awareness - as in the experience of what you're eating. Your mind will gradually learn how to make you eat less because you're helping your mind to register how and what you have just eaten.

This is an example of the Food Emotional Note; "I just ate a plate (around 50 grams) of brown rice and I felt it was cooked fine, not much salt but I enjoyed that amount. I also ate a green apple. I felt a good crunch in each bite, it was sweet, not sugary and a nice taste of sour, over all I enjoyed its taste and one apple was enough". That's just an example, and in that way you're teaching your mind to register the foods you're eating, and you're enhancing the sense of your awareness. I assure you, whenever you start doing this technique, you will start to enjoy your food more because you are appreciating the food through your senses consciously. This will also activate other positive awareness within you and will lead you to appreciate more things in your life in general. 99% of people who I taught this technique have achieved great results in regards to their weight issues. If they could do it, I believe you also can do it too.

Making your house safe and diseases free

First of all, you have to get rid of any sugary beverages such as soda drinks, sweet drinks (even the diet, light, zero sugar), energy drinks, sports drinks, and that includes the fruit juice you buy from supermarkets. There are no vitamins in that juice, and you don't need those little amounts of vitamins from that juice because you can get them from somewhere else such as "real fruits". The bottled juice you buy contains very low to zero natural juice content. And also contains very high amount of sugar, which is sometimes even higher than the normal soda drinks. On the other hand, choosing diet drinks or zero sugar drinks which contain aspartame isn't a better choice. Some people drink zero sugar drinks because they think they will lose weight, but actually, it makes you gain weight (as well as getting other health issues) because it makes you hyperglasimic and so you tend to eat, snack and nibble – and so you gain weight.

Nonetheless, you need to keep the insulin level down. It is one of the most important factors in weight issues. It causes lack of Laptin signaling and functions; the best way to do that is to get more dietary fiber in your food! You must have the carbohydrate with fiber because that will reduce the insulin response. Your insulin will not go high because your blood sugar won't go high, and the way you do it is by looking at the back of the food package or product where you can read the "Nutrition Information". You look at where it says "Dietary Fiber" and you need minimum 3 grams of fiber or higher per serving.

Another thing you need to keep away from home is MSG especially if it's combined with aspartame, such as having potato chips with soda drink! Lots of companies hide MSG when labelling their products behind the code of (E 621 / 622). There are numerous of studies show the risks when combining those two exotoxins "aspartame and MSG" and their reverse effects on behavior leading to violent behavior especially with young adults.

Excitotoxins are substances in foods that overstimulate neuron receptors in the brain and damage brain cells. These neurons then become exhausted and die. Scientists have especially noted this effect in the hypothalamus, the part of the brain that modulates behavior, impulse control, the onset of puberty, sleep and immunity. Headaches are the most common side effect. The main two excitotoxins are monosodium glutamate (MSG) and aspartame, an artificial sweetener, also called Equal or NutraSweet.

Symptoms of MSG ingestion can mimic allergic reactions, such as rashes, wheals on the skin, swollen face, hives, asthma, runny nose, flushing, rapid heartbeat, diarrhea, stomach cramps and arthritis. Neurological symptoms include depression, insomnia, anxiety, confusion and paranoia. MSG has also been linked in scientific studies to death of brain tissue in lab animals, obesity, reproductive disorders, behavioral disorders, hyperglycemia, learning and memory disorders, stroke, epilepsy, brain trauma and schizophrenia.

The general rule is that the more processed a food is, the more MSG it contains. Canned soups, soup mixes, potato chips, crackers, soy sauce, infant formula, vaccines, some wines, protein bars, dietary supplements, and especially soy products contain MSG. When a food contains less than 99 percent MSG, the ingredient does not require a label. However, hydrolyzed vegetable protein must be on the label and that always contains MSG. "Flavors" and "natural flavoring" are probable sources of MSG.

Believe it or not, conventional fruits and vegetables can be sources of MSG! A product called Auxi-Gro, which contains MSG, is sprayed on crops such as wine grapes as a growth enhancer, and MSG can end up in supposedly healthy fruits and vegetables. Organic fruits and vegetables are less likely to be sprayed with Auxi-Gro.

Fast foods and processed foods are loaded with excitotoxins and should not be consumed, especially by growing children. Cooking homemade meals from simple basic ingredients is the solution to avoiding most excitotoxins at home. MSG and its evil twin aspartame are the darlings of the food industry because they enhance the flavor of foods, thus making relatively tasteless processed foods more flavorful and addictive.

The artificial sweetener aspartame is found in many products, from soda to candy to flavored yoghurt to beer. Parents, unaware of aspartame's damaging effects on the growing brain, may buy food products containing aspartame if weight control is an issue in the household.

The FDA lists more than ninety symptoms of aspartame toxicity, even rashes, cramps and pain in the tendons and ligaments. Documented neurological events include vertigo, ringing in the ears, headaches and depression. Aspartame releases methanol upon heating and digestion, and methanol poisoning causes headaches, behavioral disturbances and inflammation of the nerves. Another breakdown product of aspartame is poisonous formaldehyde, the same substance used by undertakers to preserve corpses.

Aspartame is composed of two amino acids, aspartic acid and phenylalanine. Seizures and other mental symptoms associated with aspartame consumption are related to low serotonin resulting from the phenylalanine component. Aspartic acid is synthesized from glutamate, a major excitatory transmitter in the brain. A lack of the calming neurotransmitter serotonin and increased levels of an excitatory transmitter further stimulate the brain.

Thousands of adverse reactions to aspartame have been reported to the FDA, mostly concerned with abnormal brain function, brain tumors, epilepsy and Parkinson's disease. Children's brains are four times more susceptible to damage from excitotoxins than the brains of adults, and they react with ADD-ADHD-type symptoms, impaired learning, depression and nausea.

The USDA recently condemned sugary soda drinks for school lunch programs but considers artificially sweetened beverages a "healthier" choice.

Neurological damage from excitotoxins also depends on the quality of the diet. Those who eat antioxidant-rich foods such as organic colorful fruits and vegetables, high-quality protein and good fats such as butter, lard, coconut oil and others, are protected from the occasional food containing MSG. Cod liver oil and turmeric can reduce the likelihood of damage.

The healthy way to eat

As I mentioned earlier, many people tend to eat without knowing what and how much they are eating, especially if they are hungry. It's recommended to wait at least 20 minutes for your second meal or portion. Also, parents should apply this with their children. If a child is still hungry, teach them to wait for 20 minutes before you make the second plate for them, and that will not make you any less of a parent. This is how it works - according to the National Center for Biotechnology Information, U.S. National Library of Medicine, there is a hunger hormone in the stomach called ghrelin. When the stomach is empty ghrelin goes up and sends a message to the brain indicating that you're hungry. When you eat, ghrelin level will start to decline. However, this is not the end because the reduction of ghrelin ends up reducing hunger, but it doesn't cause or induce the feeling of satiety (the state of feeling full). Hunger and satiety are two different things. Satiety comes at the end of the intestine and the way it works is; the food goes in the stomach, the food has to cross 22 feet in the intestine. Then moving through the muscles of the intestine (which are called Peristalsis), it then gets to the end of the intestines, where specific cells in the intestine release a hormone called "peptide", which circulates in the blood stream and goes to your brain. The signal tells your hypothalamus (the department in your brain which controls eating) that you've had enough food and you're full, and the meal is over! So, it takes 20 feet of intestine to get that satiety or feeling full signal. This is why you need to wait for at least 20 minutes for the second plate or second meal portion. It gives a chance for the food to work! Also when your food contains high fiber, it will help the food to move even faster than 20 minutes in the intestine, and that will cause you to get the satiety signal sooner, and also will save you the second portion calories, fat, carbs, and the rest.

Intermittent Fasting

I'll leave this one for you to look it up, and you ask your doctor about it. It's basically a set of effective fasting strategies which allow you to choose a certain fasting strategy that fits you and your life style. The Intermittent Fasting consists of eating between a specific window period in a day or fasts on certain day/s during the week depending on the strategy you follow.

Be aware how you read the nutritional information

It's very important to learn how to read the label on food products and to know the quality and quantity the product contains in its nutrition and ingredients.

However, the nutritional information details which are placed usually at the back of food packages can be misleading sometimes.

Let's use for example a packet or bag of potato chips; it is claimed that it contains "10g of carbohydrates per serving", which is true for an average bag of potato chips, but you need to read how much is the serving according to company's calculations. You'll find their serving size is 20g - which is only 10 chips! That means every one chip contains 2g of carbs!

The real question is; are you really going to eat only 10 chips from that junk bag? Usually, an average person will eat around 70 – 100g per serving not as they state (10 chips), that's 100g of bad carbs you get from snacking on a bag of junk which will make you more hungry later and has no nutritional value whatsoever! That also goes with calories on the packets; the same bag of chips claims 590kj per their serving (141cal), but the fact is you'll end up eating the 100g which is almost 2200kj (526cal), that's almost 90 minutes of running on the treadmill with medium level intensity to be able to burn them off.

This is how you should calculate it; if a bag of potato chips is 200g net weight, and you know you're going to eat half of that bag, it means you have to calculate you're eating 100g serving, not what they claim "20g". The reason they show you smaller numbers (amount per serving) is to deceive your mind with the smaller numbers of calories, fats, and carbs, to make you think this product is not so bad, and also to make you buy it.

In addition and regarding potato chips, notice that you usually have the ability to eat a whole entire bag of potato chips without even noticing, because chips have a "vanishing choleric density". Which means, it tricks our tongue and brain into thinking that you haven't actually eaten anything. That explains the reason why the amount of "per serve" which the company claim isn't effective or accurate. 10 chips is the serving portion which most companies place on their products is not even close to a logical reality.

Also, another thing worth mentioning regarding how manufactures deceive people with label packages. Let's take for example a bag of bread, typically conscious consumers know that whole-meal, whole wheat or brown bread which is high in fiber would be a healthier choice than white bread. However, what they don't know is some bread labelled as whole wheat are nothing more than white bread with food coloring added. Bread manufactures know that more customers are moving toward wheat bread for the health benefits are associated with it. Therefore, bread companies make claims as they include whole wheat or whole grains. But that brown rich color is just a dye color to make people think it's because this bread is whole wheat and grains.

By law, the labels on foods must list the ingredients by weight but the manufacture can still put whole grain on the packaging label even if it's just a pinch of whole wheat flower or grains.

Therefore, don't be deceived next time you buy bread and look at the label for added fake brown coloring and how much whole wheat the bread contains by weight not by color.

The point is, many products are labeled to deceive people and many products are manufactured to appear healthy to deceive consumers for profit reasons. Conscious buying isn't only to buy organic products, but also to know what you're buying consciously.

Exercise

The benefits of exercise go far beyond weight management and physical appearance. Many researches show that regular physical activity can help reduce the risks for several diseases and health conditions and also improve the overall quality of one's life. Regular physical activity can help protect you from many health problems.

For instance, a 30-minute walk every day can do more for your long-term health than all the efforts of a dozen doctors and their medications.

According to Dr. William Kraus, associate professor of medicine at Duke University Medical Centre, in an article published in The New England Journal of Medicine, stated: "Even a moderate amount of exercise helps your heart. Some exercise is better than none and more is better than less." There are many benefits from exercising besides cleansing your body and keeping you young and fit. Those benefits are for you, and when you exercise you're rewarding yourself with those benefits such as maintaining the health of your heart, preventing osteoporosis (bone diseases), lowering high blood pressure, reducing stress, reducing the severity of asthma, reducing diabetic complications, promoting a healthy pregnancy, preventing cancers, promoting a healthy brain, promoting a better sex life, improving impotence (males sexual dysfunction or maintain an erection), improving sleeping patterns, helps in preventing strokes, improving oxygen and nutrient supply to all cells in your body, improving muscle strength, joint structure and joint function, helps to manage arthritis and the list goes on.

My personal experience from self-experiments

Note, the following is based on my personal experiments on myself, and please keep in mind that the same effective formula might not work for everyone.

My first and most important advice are to stop drinking any type of beverages, juices, energy drinks and any drink that contains sugar or sweeteners, even if it claims that it contains vitamins. Always go with the fresh juice you make at home if you're concerned about vitamins. I got rid of almost 5 pounds (2.3 kg) in the first 5 weeks when I stopped drinking these beverages. I replaced it all with water and felt many changes physically and psychologically.

Also, reduce the amount of sugar and salt in your food. If you're having a cup of tea and you put two spoons of sugar, try to reduce it to one, and then none. It might not taste as it used to in the beginning because you are used to the fake sweet taste. You'll soon get used to the sugarless taste, and you won't be adding any sugar to your tea after you detox. Keep in mind, everything we do is based on habits, including tastes, because they are nothing but anchors and programs in our minds. You can reduce those habits by first acknowledging them, and then do something about them. There is another bonus when you cut on the salt and sugar in your food. You will start to appreciate the real flavor of the food, especially the healthy foods.

Lastly, exercise. Exercise isn't only going to the gym, you can walk every day for 30 minutes while listening to audio-books, music or whatever keeps you motivated. No matter where you are or what you do, you can always invest some time in your health and well-being. At the end, it's your health, and you're worth it. You deserve the healthy life just as everybody else does. Remember how important and unique you are, especially because there is only one of you, and that is you!

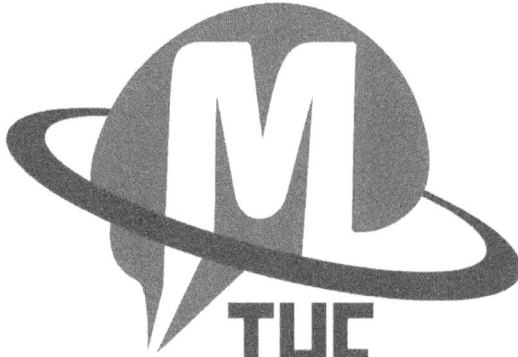

THE
MINDTECH
INSTITUTE

www.themindtechinstitute.com
www.mti.edu.au

Few Last Words

I would like to forward my sincere apologies to you, my dear reader if I've offended you in any way, because that's not what I intended to do. I tried my best to keep this book as scientific as I could, as you may have observed when reading the book. I wrote this book in a "based on and according to" format. I'm not a medical doctor or nutritional doctor, nor do I claim to be. I'm just a humble researcher in the field of sociology who happened to lecture about psychology, social science, humans' behavior and other related subjects. I also teach and run training programs with my beloved wife Denise Sivilay Musselli at our institute "The MindTech Institute".

I was reluctant in the beginning to write such a book because it's not within my professional field, and also I was in the middle of writing another book about human behaviors and social influences. However, what drove me to take the initiative to write this book is the diseases and other illnesses I've been witnessing related to foods and our lifestyle in general. While I was writing this book, specifically the chapter "Cancer – Conventional Vs Alternative Cancer Treatments", my step mother of 52 years old had passed away from cancer and obesity-related issues. It was sad but it was also expected. Sadly, because I have witnessed too many deaths of friends and others caused specifically by cancers, diabetes and other overweight related diseases in the last two decades. I have also thought of my parents and their health history, and as I always say: some parents will pass on to you their fortune, and some parents will pass on to you their medical history. I believe this is a message that I have always carried on my shoulders, until I realized that there is no better time than now to share this message with the world, hoping it will make a difference. When I read the quote of Albert Einstein "The world is a dangerous place to live, not because of the people who are evil, but because of the people who don't do anything about it", I was encouraged to be among those who do something about it. I believe that knowledge is a treasure, and keeping it away from others is a form of greed and selfishness. Therefore, I decided to share this knowledge with you as well as the world, so everyone could benefit from it.

Acknowledgement & Appreciation

Dear reader,

Lots of efforts, time, and resources were invested in this awareness project to be successfully fulfilled. However, I'm fully aware that nothing is perfect, including this book and myself. Therefore, no matter how many times I pass a book to editors and read it myself over and over again, we'll always find glitches, errors, typos mistakes and other errors. Nonetheless, I believe it's a good thing - because that's how we evolve and get better at what we do! When I was writing this book I focused more on delivering a fruitful message, rather than presenting some fancy language. And I'm glad that I did my best to deliver to you the best I could. Therefore, I urge you to share whatever knowledge you have learnt from this book with others. We can always be among those who will do something about it.

Adam Musselli

And always keep in mind that

"The world is a dangerous place to live; not because of the people who are evil, but because of the people who don't do anything about it."

- Albert Einstein

Special Thanks

I owe a special word of gratitude to my beloved wife Denise Sivilay Musselli for being supportive, encouraging and such a great blessing in my life. I am also indebted to my dear friend Dr. Alfredo Belen Sese, a veterinarian surgeon, for providing me with personal and face to face assistance in writing the chapter "Depressed Animals = Depressed Humans".

Another special word of gratitude and appreciation to our main editors in Sydney Australia for always being a great support to The MindTech Institute and for the excellent work they provide especially in editing and proofreading our publications.

I also thank all the professionals and the universities, institutes, organizations who shared their research and work with me to complete this project. And for all those who I forgot to mention, and to everyone who supported this book in its publication.

The biggest thanks are to you my dear reader, and I hope that you found what you were seeking.

About The Author

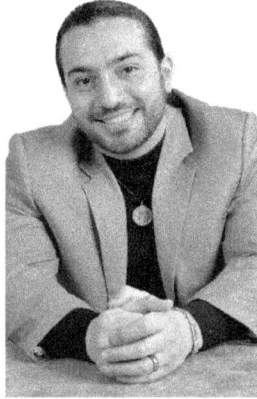

Adam Musselli

Adam has been in the field of psychology, social science and research for more than 15 years.

Adam's educational, experience, multi-lingual background as well as understanding human's behavior, sociology and psychology has given him a broad base from which to approach many topics. He believes knowledge is an essential element to life just as food and air, and he also believes in the simplicity of training and teaching as he always quotes "If you can't explain it simply, you don't understand it well enough." - Albert Einstein.

Adam is the founder and a director of The MindTech Institute. He runs several seminars, workshops and courses in Australia and globally throughout the year as well as through www.themindtechinstitute.com and www.mti.edu.au

Adam also covers various topics on his podcast "The Dynamic Thinking Project Podcast" which is available on iTunes, YouTube as well as all the major podcast platforms and other media broadcast outlets.

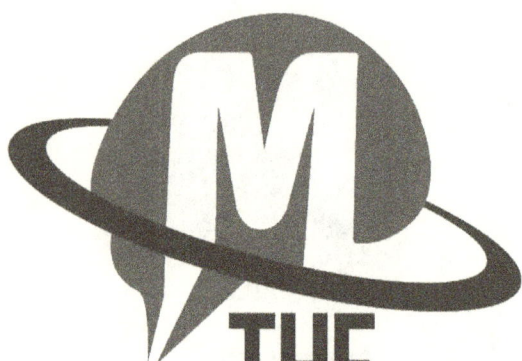

THE
MINDTECH
INSTITUTE

www.themindtechinstitute.com
www.mti.edu.au

Notes

Introduction

1- CDC, "More than one-third (36.5% or 79.6 million) of U.S. adults are obese," Centers for Disease Control (CDC), September 1, 2016, https://www.cdc.gov/obesity/data/adult.html.

2- JAMA, "The estimated annual medical cost of obesity in the U.S. was $147 billion USD...," Journal of American Medicine (JAMA), February 26, 2014, Vol 311, No. 8, http://jama.jamanetwork.com/article.aspx?articleid=1832542.

3- Albert Einstein, "The world is a dangerous place to live; not because...," Prof. Daniel Palanker, Stanford University, http://web.stanford.edu/~palanker/wisdom.html.

Chapter 1

1. Barry M. Popkin, Linda S. Adair, and Shu Wen Ng, "The Global Nutrition Transition," US National Library of Medicine National Institutes of Health, 2012 Jan; 70(1): 3–21, http://www.ncbi.nlm.nih.gov/pmc/articles/PMC3257829/.

2. The University of Utah, "A Grassy Trend in Human Ancestors' Diets," June 3, 2013, http://archive.unews.utah.edu/news_releases/a-grassy-trend-in-human-ancestors-diets/.

3. Authoritative information and statistics to promote better health and wellbeing, "3 in 5 Australian's are overweight or obese," 2011–12 Australian Bureau of Statistics Australian Health Survey, http://www.aihw.gov.au/overweight-and-obesity/.

4. Gatineau Mary, Hancock Caroline, Holman Naomi, Outhwaite Helen, Oldridge Lorraine, Christie Anna and Ells Louisa, "62% of adults were overweight or obese in England," Public Health England, July 2014, https://www.gov.uk/government/uploads/system/uploads/attachment_data/file/338934/Adult_obesity_and_type_2_diabetes_.pdf, p7.

5. The Centers for Disease Control and Prevention (CDC),"70.7% of adults age 20 years and over with overweight, including

obesity," 2013 – 1014,
http://www.cdc.gov/nchs/fastats/obesity-overweight.htm.
6.   Worldwatch Institute, "nearly two billion people worldwide now are overweight," June 14, 2011, http://www.worldwatch.org/nearly-two-billion-people-worldwide-now-overweight.

Chapter 2

1.   Joshua Freeman, "protest against high food prices," American Empire: The Rise of a Global Power, the Democratic Revolution at Home, 1945-2000 (The Penguin History of the United States), August 6 2013, Penguin Books, chap. 11 p 486.
2.   Robbins, William (4 October 1976). "Butz Delights in Conflict". Lakeland Ledger via New York Times. Retrieved 9 June 2015.
3.   Jack Ralph Kloppenburg, "either get big or get out, grow or go", "adapt or die", First the Seed: The Political Economy of Plant Biotechnology, 1492-2000, University of Wisconsin Press; 2 edition (March 16, 2005), p 136.
4.   Hanover LM, White JS (1993). "Manufacturing, composition, and applications of fructose". Am J Clin Nutr. 58 (suppl 5): 724S–732S.
5.   Bray GA, Nielsen SJ, Popkin BM, "Obesity is a major epidemic, but its causes are still unclear," Am J Clin Nutr. 2004 Apr;79(4):537-43, http://www.ncbi.nlm.nih.gov/pubmed/15051594.
6.   Jorge Fernandez-Cornejo, Seth Wechsler, Mike Livingston, and Lorraine Mitchell, "Monsanto 90% of the GE seeds planted globally in 2003," Economic Research Report Number 162 February 2014, http://www.ers.usda.gov/media/1282246/err162.pdf.
7.   Jordan Wilkerson, Brian Chow, "Roundup Ready will survive Monsanto's glyphosate herbicide while killing everything else around it", AUGUST 10, 2015, http://sitn.hms.harvard.edu/flash/2015/roundup-ready-crops/.

Chapter 3

1. GM Science Review First Report, "G.M.O stands for Genetically Modified Organisms and G.E. stands for Genetically Engineered.," Prepared by the UK GM Science Review panel (July 2003). Chairman Professor Sir David King, Chief Scientific Advisor to the UK Government, P 9

2. Megan L. Norris, "GMO food causes infertility, holes in the gastrointestinal tract (GI tract), damages organs, immune system failure, multiple organ system failure and accelerates aging.," AUGUST 10, 2015, http://sitn.hms.harvard.edu/flash/2015/will-gmos-hurt-my-body/.

3. Ari Levaux, "Chinese researchers show that microscopic RNA," JAN 9, 2012, http://www.theatlantic.com/health/archive/2012/01/the-very-real-danger-of-genetically-modified-foods/251051/.

4. World Health Organization (WHO), "organisms of which their genetic material (DNA) has been altered in such a way that it does not occur naturally," May 5 2010, http://www.who.int/foodsafety/areas_work/food-technology/faq-genetically-modified-food/en/.

5. Nutr Rev, "The FDA's 1992 policy statement granted genetically engineered foods presumptive GRAS (generally recognized as safe) status," 2005 Jun;63(6 Pt 1), http://www.ncbi.nlm.nih.gov/pubmed/16028565.

6. Prof. Ric Bessin, Extension Entomologist, "Within minutes, the protein binds to the gut wall and the insect stops feeding…," ENTFACT-130: Bt-Corn - What It Is and How It Works, University of Kentucky College of Agriculture, https://entomology.ca.uky.edu/ef130.

7. Eur J Pediatr, "BT toxin was detected in the bloodstream of 69% of the population…," 2006 Nov; 165(Suppl 1): 1–389., http://www.ncbi.nlm.nih.gov/pmc/articles/PMC2799065/.

8. Nina Kraft, "Åshild Krogdahl matched two groups of animals such as rats, mice…," July 11 2012, http://forskning.no/genmodifisert-mat/2012/07/rotter-fetere-av-genmat.

9. Bakke-McKellep, A.M., Koppang, E.O., Gunnes, G., Sanden, M., Hemre, G.I., Landsverk, T., Krogdahl, A., 2007." the ones who had fed on GM corn were slightly larger…," Histological, digestive, metabolic,

hormonal and some immune factor responses in Atlantic salmon, Salmo salar L., fed genetically modified soybeans. Journal of Fish Diseases 30, 65-79, http://sciencenordic.com/growing-fatter-gm-diet.

10. Amy M. Branum, M.S.P.H. and Susan L. Lukacs, D.O., M.S.P.H., "Food Allergy Among U.S. Children: Trends in Prevalence and Hospitalizations," 10, October 2008, http://www.cdc.gov/nchs/products/databriefs/db10.htm.

11. National Institute of Allergy and Infectious Diseases, "The first time you are exposed to a food allergen…," U.S. DEPARTMENT OF HEALTH AND HUMAN SERVICES, National Institutes of Health (NIAID, NIH), NIH Publication No. 12-5518, July 2012, https://www.niaid.nih.gov/topics/foodallergy/documents/foodallergy .pdf.

12. Marty Pearce, Brian Habbick, Janice Williams, Margaret Eastman, Maureen Newman, "a bacterial pest control product called Foray 48B…," Canadian Journal Of Public Health, January – February 2002, P 21, https://extension.entm.purdue.edu/GM/PDF/GMquestions.

13. Dr. Phylis B. Canion, "several animal studies indicate serious health risks associated with genetically modified foods," AuthorHouse, Read All About It: Q's & A's About Nutrition, Volume 3, July 6 2013, P 71.

14. Food & Water Watch, "the food and agriculture biotechnology industry has spent more than $572 million in campaign contributions and lobbying expenses," November 2010, P 1, https://www.foodandwaterwatch.org/sites/default/files/Biotech%20L obbying%20IB%20Nov%202010_0.pdf.

15. Genetic Literacy Project, "Scientists react to republished Séralini GMO maize rat study," June 24, 2014, Genetic Literacy Project, www.geneticliteracyproject.org/2014/06/24/scientists-react-to-republished-seralini-maize-rat-study/.

16. Michael K. Hansen, Ph.D., "Dr. Hansen explains in an interview with Steve Curwood," December 6, 2013, loe.org.

Chapter 4

1. The Staff Of The Select Committee On Nutrition And Human Needs, "Dietary Goals for United States," United States Senate in 95th Congress, 1st session in February 1977, p 12 section 2.

2. U.S. Food and Drug Administration, "Aspartame," CFSAN/Office of Food Additive Safety, April 20, 2007, http://www.fda.gov/Food/IngredientsPackagingLabeling/FoodAdditiv esIngredients/ucm208580.htm.

3. Dr. Nibodhi Haas, Gunavati Gobbi, "there are over 92 different health side effects associated with aspartame consumption," Ayurvedic Nutrition, Mata Amritanandamayi Mission Trust, p 45.

4. Mariana Verdelho Machado, Helena Cortez-Pinto, "fatty liver disease non-alcoholic which now affects one third of all Americans," World J Gastroenterol. 2014 Sep 28; 20(36): 12956–12980, National Center for Biotechnology Information, U.S. National Library of Medicine, http://www.ncbi.nlm.nih.gov/pmc/articles/PMC4177476/.

5. Esther Eisenberg, M.D., M.P.H., "Polycystic Ovarian Syndrome now affects 10% in all women," Polycystic ovary syndrome (PCOS) fact sheet, December 23, 2014, the Office on Women's Health in the Office of the Assistant Secretary for Health at the U.S. Department of Health and Human Services, http://womenshealth.gov/publications/our-publications/fact-sheet/polycystic-ovary-syndrome.html.

6. Cheryl Fryar, M.S.P.H., Cynthia Ogden, Ph.D., M.R.P, "20% of obese people have a totally normal cellular metabolism…," The National Institute of Diabetes and Digestive and Kidney Diseases, Overweight and Obesity Statistics, October 2012, https://www.niddk.nih.gov/health-information/health-statistics/Pages/overweight-obesity-statistics.aspx.

7. United Nations, "non-communicable disease that chronic, metabolic disease…," GA/11138, 19 SEPTEMBER 2011, Sixty-sixth General Assembly, 3rd, 4th & 5thMeetings, http://www.un.org/press/en/2011/ga11138.doc.htm.

8. Priya Rajagopalan, Arthur W. Toga, Clifford R. Jack, Michael W. Weiner, Paul M. Thompson, "Leptin, a hormone produced by body fat tissue," National Center for Biotechnology Information, U.S. National Library of Medicine, Neuroreport. 2013 Jan 23; 24(2): 58–62, doi: 10.1097/WNR.0b013e32835c5254, http://www.ncbi.nlm.nih.gov/pmc/articles/PMC3635486/.

9. Gilberto Paz-Filho, Claudio Mastronardi, Ma-Li Wong, Julio Licinio, "Researchers have found a very significant answer to the reason that causes Leptin Resistance," National Center for Biotechnology Information, U.S. National Library of Medicine, 2012 Dec; 16(Suppl 3): S549–S555, http://www.ncbi.nlm.nih.gov/pmc/articles/PMC3602983/.

10. Prof. Robert H. Lustig, "You are an average healthy person. You eat 2000 calories a day and you burn 2000 calories...," University of California, San Francisco UCSF, http://www.uctv.tv/shows/The-Skinny-on-Obesity-Ep-1-An-Epidemic-for-Every-Body-23305.

11. Marie Amitani, Akihiro Asakawa, Haruka Amitani, Akio Inui, "The role of leptin in the control of insulin-glucose axis," National Center for Biotechnology Information, U.S. National Library of Medicine, 2013 Apr 8. doi: 10.3389/fnins.2013.00051, http://www.ncbi.nlm.nih.gov/pmc/articles/PMC3619125/.

12. NIH, "Dopamine," NIH U.S. National Library of Medicine National Center for Biotechnology Information, 2004-09-16, https://pubchem.ncbi.nlm.nih.gov/compound/dopamine#section=Top.

13. Nicole M. Avena, Pedro Rada, Bartley G. Hoebel, "sugar down-regulates the same receptors in the reward center," US National Library of Medicine National Institutes of Health, 2008; 32(1): 20–39., http://www.ncbi.nlm.nih.gov/pmc/articles/PMC2235907/.

14. Martin JA, Hamilton BE, Sutton PD, "women gained 40 lbs. (18.1 kg) since 1990 to 2005 is 20%," National Vital Statistics System. Annual natality files, final data for 2005. Natl Vital Stat Rep 2007; 56 (6), Centers for Disease Control and Prevention CDC, http://www.cdc.gov/mmwr/preview/mmwrhtml/mm5705a7.htm.

15. The American Academy of Child and Adolescent Psychiatry Studies, "a child who is obese between the ages of 10 and 13 has an 80 percent chance of becoming obese as an adult." No. 79; April 2016, http://www.aacap.org/AACAP/Families_and_Youth/Facts_for_Families/FFF-Guide/Obesity-In-Children-And-Teens-079.aspx.

16. The National Heart Foundation of Australia, "Refined carbohydrate foods are highly processed with little or no wholegrain fiber," Feb 2006 National Heart Foundation of Australia PP-584, p 11,

https://www.heartfoundation.org.au/images/uploads/publications/C arbohydrates-dietary-fibre-QA.pdf.
17. Nutrition and Your Health, "more than 60 percent of our foods should be in the form of complex carbohydrates," Dietary Guidelines for Americans, fifth edition, 2000.
18. According to Minnesota Department of Health MDH, "whole grain kernel consists of 3 parts," October 08, 2014, http://www.health.state.mn.us/divs/hpcd/chp/cdrr/nutrition/facts/w holegrains.html.

Chapter 5

1. Elaine Magee, MPH, RD, "Children's Hospital in Boston, teens aged 13 - 17 were given three types of fast-food meals," Junk-Food Facts, p 1, http://documents.tips/documents/junk-foods-56b1e8b10e424.html.
2. Jessica Anderson, RD, "The body can only handle so much at one time," Amanda Gardner, http://www.health.com/health/gallery/0,,20551987,00.html#high-fat-and-fried-food.
3. Center for Science in the Public Interest, "About Trans Fat and Partially Hydrogenated Oils," https://en.wikipedia.org/wiki/Center_for_Science_in_the_Public_Inte rest.
4. Russell L. Blaylock, MD, "The Taste that kills," Volume 38, No. 1, http://americannutritionassociation.org/newsletter/review-excitotoxins-taste-kills.
5. Dr. David Ludwig, MD, PhD, "Almost 1/3rd of the children in the United States eat fast food regularly…," CBS News, Jaime Holguin, January 5, 2004, http://www.cbsnews.com/news/fast-food-linked-to-child-obesity/.
6. Emily Wax, RD, The Brooklyn Hospital Center, Brooklyn, NY., David Zieve, MD, MHA, Isla Ogilvie, PhD, A.D.A.M. Editorial team, "Heart disease, heart attacks, and stroke," Heart disease and diet, Heart disease and diet, MedicinePlus, last updated April 25 2015, https://medlineplus.gov/ency/article/002436.htm#top.
7. Department of Health & Human Services, Deakin University, "Heart disease and food," The Department of Health & Human Services, State

Government of Victoria, Australia, September 2012, https://www.betterhealth.vic.gov.au/health/conditionsandtreatments/heart-disease-and-food.

8. Cancer Council NSW, "nitrites carcinogenic...," Cancer Council NSW, http://www.cancercouncil.com.au/86049/cancer-information/general-information-cancer-information/cancer-questions-myths/food-and-drink/food-preservatives-do-not-cause-cancer/.

9. National Toxicology Program, Department of Health and Human Services," N-Nitrosamines," Report on Carcinogens, Thirteenth Edition, https://ntp.niehs.nih.gov/ntp/roc/content/profiles/nitrosamines.pdf.

10. Mark Russell, "'Fresh' meat stored weeks or months," Sydney Morning Harold, January 30 2011, http://www.smh.com.au/national/fresh-meat-stored-weeks-or-months-20110129-1a8xn.html.

11. About Food & Water Watch, "2004 the FDA approved injecting meat with carbon monoxide...," About Food & Water Watch, April 2008, https://www.foodandwaterwatch.org/sites/default/files/carbon_monoxide_report_apr_2008.pdf.

12. Ohnishi M, Razzaque MS. "Dietary and genetic evidence for phosphate toxicity accelerating mammalian aging," the Federation of American Societies for Experimental Biology FASEB, US National Library of Medicine, National Institutes of Health, 2010 Sep; 24(9):3562-71, http://www.ncbi.nlm.nih.gov/pubmed/20418498.

13. Shawkat Razzaque, M.D., Ph.D., "Phosphate toxicity: new insights into an old problem," US National Library of Medicine, National Institutes of Health, Clin Sci (Lond). 2011 Feb; 120(3): 91–97., http://www.ncbi.nlm.nih.gov/pmc/articles/PMC3120105/.

14. Gerald Weissmann, M.D., "High levels of phosphate in sodas...," ScienceDaily, April 28, 2010, Federation of American Societies for Experimental Biology, https://www.sciencedaily.com/releases/2010/04/100426151636.htm.

15. McGinnis JM, Foege WH., "Actual causes of death in the United States." JAMA 1993; 270:2207-12.

16. World Health Organization, ""About diabetes," 4 April 2014, http://www.who.int/diabetes/action_online/basics/en/.

17. USCB, "The world population in 2013," http://www.census.gov/popclock/.
18. Lancet, Harvard College ", 347 million adults in the world have diabetes," June 25, 2011, https://www.hsph.harvard.edu/news/press-releases/diabetes-global-epidemic/.
19. IDF, "387 million people have diabetes; by 2035 this will rise to 592 million", International Diabetes Federation (IDF), Key Findings 2014, http://www.idf.org/diabetesatlas/update-2014.
20. Australian Institute of Health and Welfare, "480,000 children in the world live with diabetes," Aug 5, 2010, http://www.aihw.gov.au/WorkArea/DownloadAsset.aspx?id=6442455124.
21. Andrew O. Odegaard, Woon Puay Koh, Jian-Min Yuan, Myron D. Gross, Mark A. Pereira, "that people who consume fast food two or more times a week were found to increase the risk of developing Type 2 diabetes by 27%," the American Heart Association's journal Circulation, July 10, 2012, http://circ.ahajournals.org/content/126/2/182.
22. American Diabetes Association, "cost of diagnosed diabetes in 2012 is $245 billion," Economic Costs of Diabetes in the U.S. in 2012, 2013 Mar; DC_122625., http://care.diabetesjournals.org/content/early/2013/03/05/dc12-2625.
23. Laura Hughes, "£16 billion pounds is spent every year on treating diabetes and its complications," The Telegraph, 7 June 2016, http://www.telegraph.co.uk/news/2016/06/07/more-spent-on-treating-obesity-related-conditions-than-on-the-po/.
24. ONS, "UK Population 2015," Office for National Statistics, June 30 2015, https://www.ons.gov.uk/peoplepopulationandcommunity/populationandmigration/populationestimates.
25. ABS, "Australia Population 2014," the Australian Bureau of Statistics, December 31 2015 http://www.abs.gov.au/ausstats/abs@.nsf/0/1647509ef7e25faaca2568a900154b63?opendocument.

26. AusDiab, "diabetes type two annual spending," The Australian Diabetes, Obesity and Lifestyle study AusDiab, 2012, https://www.bakeridi.edu.au/Assets/Files/Baker%20IDI%20Aus diab%20Report_interactive_FINAL.pdf.

27. IDF, "Global diabetes,"International Diabetes Federation IDF, 2014, http://www.diabetesatlas.org.

28. American Heart Association, "'Western' Diet Increases Heart Attack Risk Globally," October 22, 2008, ScienceDaily, https://www.sciencedaily.com/releases/2008/10/081020171337.htm.

29. J Am Coll Cardiol, "Food Consumption and its impact on Cardiovascular Disease: Importance of Solutions focused on the globalized food system," National Center for Biotechnology Information, U.S. National Library of Medicine, Oct 6 2015; 66(14): 1590–1614., http://www.ncbi.nlm.nih.gov/pmc/articles/PMC4597475/.

30. University of Las Palmas de Gran Canarias, "Link between fast food and depression confirmed," ScienceDaily, March 30, 2012, https://www.sciencedaily.com/releases/2012/03/120330081352.htm.

31. Laura Bailey, "excess sugar and fat in the body could weaken the bones and lead to osteoporosis," University of Michigan Regents Michigan News, Dec 21, 2012, http://www.ns.umich.edu/new/releases/21049-fruit-in-your-holiday-stocking-can-help-keep-bones-strong.

32. Linda K. Massey Ph.D. RD, "Not just obesity: Junk food causes osteoporosis," Ben Meredith, Natural News, January 22, 2013, http://www.naturalnews.com/038773_junk_food_osteoporosis_obes ity.html.

33. UCSF, "Chronic Stress Heightens Vulnerability to Diet-Related Metabolic Risk," Juliana Bunim, University of California San Francisco, April 29, 2014, https://www.ucsf.edu/news/2014/04/113881/chronic-stress-heightens-vulnerability-diet-related-metabolic-risk.

34. Department of Health & Human Services, State Government of Victoria, Australia, "Gallbladder and its functions," Department of Health & Human Services, State Government of Victoria, Australia, https://www.betterhealth.vic.gov.au/health/conditionsandtreatment s/gallbladder-gallstones-and-surgery.

35. National Cancer Institute, "Types of cancers," National Cancer Institute, http://www.cancer.gov/types.

36. Andy Meharg, "High levels of arsenic in rice," Independent, November 4, 2014, http://www.independent.co.uk/life-style/health-and-families/features/high-levels-of-arsenic-in-rice-why-isnt-it-regulated-in-our-food-9836900.html.

37. Agency for Toxic Substances and Disease, "Toxic Substances Portal – Arsenic," Agency for Toxic Substances and Disease, February 12, 2013, http://www.atsdr.cdc.gov/toxfaqs/tf.asp?id=19&tid=3.

38. WHO, "Frequently asked questions on genetically modified foodsWorld Health Organization (WHO), http://www.who.int/foodsafety/areas_work/food-technology/faq-genetically-modified-food/en/.

39. Cancer Research UK, "Microwave ovens don't cause cancer," http://www.cancerresearchuk.org/about-cancer/cancers-in-general/cancer-questions/radiation-microwaves-and-cancer#sIHhmdFBu4I6l8Am.99.

40. Mueller NT, Odegaard A, Anderson K, "Data Clearly Links Soda Consumption to Pancreatic Cancer," the Singapore Chinese Health Study. Cancer Epidemiol Biomarkers Prev. 2010; 19(2):447-455., Jacob Schor, ND, FABNO, March 2010 Vol. 2 Issue 3.

41. American Cancer Society, "estimated 53,070 Americans will be diagnosed with pancreatic cancer…," The 2012 edition of Cancer Facts & Figures, www.cancer.org › Explore Research › Cancer Facts and Statistics.

42. OEHHA, "4-Methylimidazole (4-MEI) A Fact Sheet," Office of Environmental Health Hazards Assessment (OEHHA), Feb 23, 2012, http://oehha.ca.gov/proposition-65/4-methylimidazole-4-mei-fact-sheet.

43. OEHHA, "Changed Notice of Proposed Rulemaking Specific Regulatory Levels Posing No Significant Risk: 4-Methylimidazole (4-MEI)," Office of Environmental Health Hazards Assessment (OEHHA), Oct 7, 2011, http://oehha.ca.gov/proposition-65/crnr/changed-notice-proposed-rulemaking-specific-regulatory-levels-posing-no.

44. Maki Inoue-Choi, PhD, MS, RD, "soda and sweet beverages and their link to cancer," NBCNEWS, Maggie Fox, NOV 22, 2013,

http://www.nbcnews.com/health/step-away-soda-sugary-drinks-raise-cancer-risk-women-study-2D11641447.
45. N. Colombo, E. Preti, F. Landoni, S. Carinelli, A. Colombo, C. Marini, C. Sessa, "Endometrial cancer," Oxford Medical Journal, Medicine & Health Annals of Oncology Volume 22, Issue suppl 6Pp. vi35-vi39.
46. Rainer J, Ulrike Kämmerer, "Is there a role for carbohydrate restriction in the treatment and prevention of cancer?," US National Library of Medicine National Institutes of Health, Oct 26, 2011, 10.1186/1743-7075-8-75,
http://www.ncbi.nlm.nih.gov/pmc/articles/PMC3267662/?tool=pubmed.
47. Jeffery A. Foran, David O. Carpenter, M. Coreen Hamilton, Barbara A. Knuth, Steven J. Schwager, "Risk-Based Consumption Advice for Farmed Atlantic and Wild Pacific Salmon Contaminated with Dioxins and Dioxin-like Compounds," US National Library of Medicine National Institutes of Health, 2005 May; 113(5): 552–556.,
http://www.ncbi.nlm.nih.gov/pmc/articles/PMC1257546/.

Chapter 6

1. Heather A. Eicher-Miller, Victor L. Fulgoni, Debra R. Keast "Contributions of Processed Foods to Dietary Intake...," US National Library of Medicine National Institutes of Health, Sep 18, 2012, doi: 10.3945/jn.112.164442,
http://www.ncbi.nlm.nih.gov/pmc/articles/PMC3593301/.
2. George Mateljan Foundation, "Some of the many additives included in processed foods are thought to have the ability to compromise the body's structure and function...," The George Mateljan Foundation, http://www.whfoods.com/genpage.php?tname=george&dbid=107.
3. Food Standards, "list of food additives" July 2014,
https://www.foodstandards.gov.au/consumer/additives/additiveoverview/Documents/Food%20Additive%20Code%20Numbers%20(July%202014).pdf.
4. USDA, "typical American household spends about 90 percent of their food budget on processed foods,"Elise Golan, Hayden Stewart, Fred Kuchler, Diansheng Dong, November 01, 2008,
http://www.ers.usda.gov/amber-waves/2008-november/can-low-income-americans-afford-a-healthy-diet.aspx#.V6_9plyOcds.

5. FDA Dockets Submittal, "Aspartame," Mark D. Gold to FDA Dockets Submittal, January 12, 2003, http://www.fda.gov/ohrms/dockets/dailys/03/jan03/012203/02p-0317_emc-000199.txt.

6. Kimber L. Stanhope,corresponding, Andrew A. Bremer, Valentina Medici, Katsuyuki Nakajima, Yasuki Ito, Takamitsu Nakano, Guoxia Chen, Tak Hou Fong, Vivien Lee, Roseanne I. Menorca, Nancy L. Keim, Peter J. Havel, "HFCS Increase Postprandial Triglycerides, LDL-Cholesterol, and Apolipoprotein-B in Young Men and Women," US National Library of Medicine National Institutes of Health, Oct 2011; 96(10): E1596–E1605., http://www.ncbi.nlm.nih.gov/pmc/articles/PMC3200248/.

7. Jennifer S. Xiong, Debbie Branigan, Minghua Li, "Deciphering the MSG controversy," US National Library of Medicine National Institutes of Health, Nov 15 2009; 2(4): 329–336., http://www.ncbi.nlm.nih.gov/pmc/articles/PMC2802046/.

8. Kummerow FA, "The negative effects of hydrogenated trans fats and what to do about them", National Library of Medicine National Institutes of Health, 2009 Aug; 205(2):458-65. doi: 10.1016/j.atherosclerosis.2009.03.009. Epub 2009 Mar 19, http://www.ncbi.nlm.nih.gov/pubmed/19345947.

9. Bernard Weiss, "Synthetic Food Colors and Neurobehavioral Hazards: The View from Environmental Health Research," National Library of Medicine National Institutes of Health, 2012 Jan; 120(1): 1–5, http://www.ncbi.nlm.nih.gov/pmc/articles/PMC3261946/.

10. Brad Olsen, "Blue #1 and Blue #2 (E133) are banned in Norway, Finland and France." Modern Esoteric: Beyond Our Senses (The Esoteric Series Book 1), CCC Publishing, March 1 2014, p 323.

11. Chiropractic Care and Longevity Center, "Red dye # 3 (also Red #40 – a more current dye) (E124)," Chiropractic Care and Longevity Center, Newsletter, September 2012, p 5.

12. Chiropractic Care and Longevity Center, "Yellow #6 (E110) and Yellow Tartrazine (E102): banned in Norway and Sweden," Chiropractic Care and Longevity Center, Newsletter, September

13. East Los Angeles College (ELAC), "Sodium Sulfite (E221)," additives to avoid,

https://www.elac.edu/academics/programs/slo/doc/Food_Additives_to_Avoid.pdf.

14. Sindelar, Jeffrey, Milkowski, Andrew, "Human safety controversies surrounding nitrate and nitrite in the diet," March 2012, Nitric Oxide. 26: 259–266. doi:10.1016/j.niox.2012.03.011.

15. Glenn Toole, Susan Toole, "hydroxyanisole)BHA (and butylated hydroxytoluese)BHT) (E 320and E321),"Nelson Thornes Ltd; New edition edition 17 Mar 1997, p 590.

16. Brad Olsen, "Sulfur Dioxide (E220): Sulfur additives are toxic. ... The International Labour Organization ofthe UN says to avoid E220 ifyou sufferfrom conjunctivitis," Modern Esoteric: Beyond Our Senses (The Esoteric Series Book 1), CCC Publishing, March 1 2014, p 324,

17. Y Kurokawa, A Maekawa, M Takahashi, Y Hayashi, "Toxicity and carcinogenicity of potassium bromate--a new renal carcinogen," ," National Library of Medicine National Institutes of Health, 1990 Jul; 87: 309–335,
http://www.ncbi.nlm.nih.gov/pmc/articles/PMC1567851/.

18. University of Southampton, "Food Standards Agency cites Southampton study in new recommendation on food additives," 10 April 2008, http://www.southampton.ac.uk/news/2008/04/food-standards-agency-cites-southampton-study.page.

19. Mamur S, Yüzbaşioğlu D, Unal F, Yilmaz S, "Does potassium sorbate induce genotoxic or mutagenic effects in lymphocytes?," ," National Library of Medicine National Institutes of Health, 2010 Apr;24(3):790-4. doi: 10.1016/j.tiv.2009.12.021. Epub 2009 Dec 2.,
https://www.ncbi.nlm.nih.gov/pubmed/20036729.

20. Nathanael Johnson, "the company can voluntarily submit its findings to the FDA" Grits, The GM safety dance: What's rule and what's real, Jul 10, 2013, http://grist.org/food/the-gm-safety-dance-whats-rule-and-whats-real/.

21. FDA spokesperson Theresa Eisenman, "it is the manufacturer's responsibility to ensure that the [GMO] food products it offers for sale are safe…," Grits, The GM safety dance: What's rule and what's real, Jul 10, 2013, http://grist.org/food/the-gm-safety-dance-whats-rule-and-whats-real/.

22. William Freese and David Schubert, "Safety Testing of Genetically Engineered Food." Biotechnology and Genetic Engineering Reviews,

November 2004, 21:299-324,
http://www.saveourseeds.org/downloads/schubert_safety_reg_us_1
1_2004.pdf.

Chapter 7

1. Medical Dictionary, "addiction definition,"   http://medical-dictionary.thefreedictionary.com/addiction
2. Nicole M. Avena, Pedro Rada, Bartley G. Hoebel, "Evidence for sugar addiction: Behavioral and neurochemical effects of intermittent, excessive sugar intake," National Library of Medicine National Institutes of Health, Neurosci Biobehav Rev. 2008; 32(1): 20–39. 18 May 2007, http://www.ncbi.nlm.nih.gov/pmc/articles/PMC2235907/.
3. Paul van der Velpen, "Sugar is 'addictive and the most dangerous drug of the times," The Telegraph, Bruno Waterfield, 17 Sep 2013, http://www.telegraph.co.uk/news/worldnews/europe/netherlands/1 0314705/Sugar-is-addictive-and-the-most-dangerous-drug-of-the-times.html.
4. The American Heart Association (AHA),"shouldn't exceed 150 calories per day...," Nov 19,2014, http://www.heart.org/HEARTORG/HealthyLiving/HealthyEating/Nutrit ion/Sugar-101_UCM_306024_Article.jsp#.V7BhyFyOcds.
5. Dr. Leri,"Addiction to unhealthy foods could help explain the global obesity epidemic," Canadian Association for Neuroscience, May 22, 2013, https://www.sciencedaily.com/releases/2013/05/130522095807.htm.
6. Dr. Leri,"We have evidence in laboratory animals of a shared vulnerability to develop preferences for sweet foods and for cocaine." Canadian Association for Neuroscience, May 22, 2013, https://www.sciencedaily.com/releases/2013/05/130522095807.htm.
7. David Kessler, "highly pleasurable. It gives you this momentary bliss. When you're eating food that is highly hedonic, it sort of takes over your brain." The Guardian, Jacques Peretti, 12 June 2012, https://www.theguardian.com/business/2012/jun/11/why-our-food-is-making-us-fat.
8. Dr. Jennifer Lee, ""Rats addicted to sugar ingest it in a binge-like manner that releases dopamine in the accumbens...," Collective

Evolution, Alanna Ketleroctober 14, 2013, http://www.collective-evolution.com/2013/10/14/sugar-is-addictive-one-of-the-most-dangerous-substances-we-consume/.

9. Department of Health and Human Services DHHS, "Today, the average American consumes almost 152 pounds (almost 69 kg) of sugar in one year…,"USDA, Department of Health and Human Services DHHS, Chapter 2, Profiling Food Consumption in America, http://www.usda.gov/factbook/chapter2.pdf

10. Duke University Medical Center, "Salt appetite is linked to drug addiction, research finds," Daily Science, July 29, 2011, https://www.sciencedaily.com/releases/2011/07/110711151451.htm.

11. Wolfgang Liedtke, M.D., Ph.D., "Our findings have profound and far-reaching medical implications…," Duke University Medical Center, Daily Science, July 29, 2011, https://www.sciencedaily.com/releases/2011/07/110711151451.htm.

12. Morris MJ, Na ES, Johnson AK., "Salt craving: the psychobiology of pathogenic sodium intake." National Library of Medicine National Institutes of Health, Physiol Behav. 2008 Aug, http://www.ncbi.nlm.nih.gov/pubmed/18514747.

13. North American Meat Institute, "Table Salt (Sodium chloride) is made of 40 percent sodium, an electrolyte that helps to maintain the fluids…," North American Meat Institute, January 2015, https://www.meatinstitute.org/index.php?ht=a/GetDocumentAction/i/93534.

14. CDC, "CDC recommends Americans consume no more than 2,300 mg of sodium per day…," National Center for Chronic Disease Prevention and Health Promotion, Division for Heart Disease and Stroke Prevention, June 1 2014, https://www.cdc.gov/salt/.

15. Journal of the American Medical Association, "Dietary Guidelines for Americans," Journal of the American Medical Association 273:404, 1995. https://health.gov/dietaryguidelines/dga95/9dietgui.htm.

16. Paul J. Kenny, Ph.D., "Fatty foods may cause cocaine-like addiction," CNN, Sarah Klein, March 30, 2010, http://edition.cnn.com/2010/HEALTH/03/28/fatty.foods.brain/.

17. Gene-Jack Wang, M.D., "Fatty foods may cause cocaine-like addiction," CNN, Sarah Klein, March 30, 2010, http://edition.cnn.com/2010/HEALTH/03/28/fatty.foods.brain/.

18. Kelly Brownell, Ph.D., "People knew for a long time cigarettes were killing people, but it was only later they learned about nicotine and the intentional manipulation of it." Bloomberg, Robert Langreth and Duane D. Stanford, November 2, 2011, http://www.bloomberg.com/news/articles/2011-11-02/fatty-foods-addictive-as-cocaine-in-growing-body-of-science.

19. Finkelstein, EA, Trogdon, JG, Cohen, JW, and Dietz, W., "Annual medical spending attributable to obesity: Payer- and service-specific estimates." National Library of Medicine National Institutes of Health, Health Affairs 2009; 28(5): w822-w831. http://www.ncbi.nlm.nih.gov/pubmed/19635784.

Chapter 8

1. Sanjay Basu, Paula Yoffe, Nancy Hills, Robert H. Lustig, "The Relationship of Sugar to Population-Level Diabetes Prevalence: An Econometric Analysis of Repeated Cross-Sectional Data," National Library of Medicine National Institutes of Health, 2013 Feb 27. doi: 10.1371/journal.pone.0057873, http://www.ncbi.nlm.nih.gov/pmc/articles/PMC3584048/.

2. Robert H. Lustig, MD, "The Diet Debacle," Project Syndicate, May 28, 2012, https://www.project-syndicate.org/commentary/the-diet-debacle.

3. Robert H. Lustig, MD, "Fructose: the poison index," The Guardian, 22 October 2013, https://www.theguardian.com/commentisfree/2013/oct/21/fructose-poison-sugar-industry-pseudoscience.

4. Johnson RK, Appel LJ, Brands M, Howard BV, Lefevre M, Lustig RH, Sacks F, Steffen LM, Wylie-Rosett J, "Dietary sugars intake and cardiovascular health: a scientific statement from the American Heart Association. National Library of Medicine National Institutes of Health, 2009 Sep 15;120(11):1011-20, http://www.ncbi.nlm.nih.gov/pubmed/19704096.

5. Robyn O'Brian, "In 1984, the largest soft drink companies replaced their sugar with corn syrup," The Huffington Post, Sep 7, 2010, http://www.huffingtonpost.com/robyn-o/why-coke-and-pepsi-should_b_707250.html.

6. Roy M. Wallack, "350 cans a year to almost 600 cans," Bike for Life: How to Ride to 100--and Beyond, Da Capo Lifelong Books; Rev Upd edition (March 10, 2015), p 112.

7. J S White, L J Hobbs, S Fernandez, "high fructose corn syrup in the sweetness index scores a 120 - 160 while sucrose is only 100," National Library of Medicine National Institutes of Health, 2015 Jan; 39(1): 176–182, http://www.ncbi.nlm.nih.gov/pmc/articles/PMC4285619/.

8. G Harvey Anderson, "HFCS has primarily been used to substitute for sucrose as a caloric sweetener," American Society for Clinical Nutrition, 2007, http://ajcn.nutrition.org/content/86/6/1577.full.

9. Pigman, Ward; Horton, D. (1972). Pigman and Horton, ed. The Carbohydrates: Chemistry and Biochemistry Vol 1A (2nd ed.). San Diego: Academic Press. pp. 1–67.

10. White JS. Sucrose, HFCS, and Fructose: History, Manufacture, Composition, Applications, and Production. Chapter 2 in J.M. Rippe (ed.), Fructose, High Fructose Corn Syrup, Sucrose and Health, Nutrition and Health. Springer Science+Business Media New York 2014.

11. S Dam-Larsen, M Franzmann, I B Andersen, P Christoffersen, L B Jensen, T I A Sørensen, U Becker, F Bendtsen, "Fatty liver is a common histological finding in human liver biopsy specimens. It affects 10–24% of the general population...," National Library of Medicine National Institutes of Health, 2004 May; 53(5): 750–755. http://www.ncbi.nlm.nih.gov/pmc/articles/PMC1774026/.

12. Dr. Dawn Irene Eshelman Singleton, PhD, "HFCS often contains toxic levels of mercury, because of color-alkali products used in its manufacturing." The Power of the Entangled Hierarchy: Never Ever Give Up, Outskirts Press, September 11, 2014, p 120.

13. Institute for Agriculture and Trade Policy, "Much High Fructose Corn Syrup Contaminated With Mercury, New Study Finds," January 26, 2009, http://www.iatp.org/documents/much-high-fructose-corn-syrup-contaminated-with-mercury-new-study-finds.

14. Lee Bracker, "HFCS arsenic, lead, chloride and heavy metals," High Frequency Food, publisher lulu, July 31, 2009, p 49.

15. Mazur, Robert H. (1974). "Aspartic acid-based sweeteners". In Inglett, George E. Symposium: sweeteners. Westport, CT: AVI Publishing. pp. 159–163.

16. Michael W. Roberts, J. Timothy Wright, "Aspartame is 220 times sweeter than sugar." National Library of Medicine National Institutes of Health, 2012 Feb 22. doi: 10.1155/2012/625701, http://www.ncbi.nlm.nih.gov/pmc/articles/PMC3296175/.

17. USDA, "Profiling Food Consumption in America - US Department of Agriculture," http://www.usda.gov/factbook/chapter2.pdf.

18. Janet Starr Hull, PhD, CN., "Aspartame Approved History," Dr. Janet Starr Hull, 2011, http://www.janethull.com/newsletter/0412/aspartame_approval_history_1.php.

19. Tom Philpott, "The Grits report," Grist, Feb 15, 2011, http://grist.org/scary-food/2011-02-14-just-how-bad-is-aspartame-the-leading-u-s-fake-sweetener/.

20. AG Nill, "FDA issued approved aspartame for use as a ...," LEDA at Harvard Law School, 2000, https://dash.harvard.edu/bitstream/handle/1/8846759/Nill,_Ashley_-_The_History_of_Aspartame.html?sequence=6.

21. Robbie Gennet, "Donald Rumsfeld and the Strange History of Aspartame," The Huffington Post, May 25, 2011, http://www.huffingtonpost.com/robbie-gennet/donald-rumsfeld-and-the-s_b_805581.html.

22. Tom Philpot, "the issue Aspartame is really not an issue of science; it's an issue of politics." Grist, Feb 15, 2011, http://grist.org/scary-food/2011-02-14-just-how-bad-is-aspartame-the-leading-u-s-fake-sweetener/.

23. Mark Gold, "Department of Health and Human Services on April 20, 1995 filed complaints and submitted to the FDA symptoms attributed to Aspartame showing over 92 different health side effects..." FDA, January 12, 2003, http://www.fda.gov/ohrms/dockets/dailys/03/jan03/012203/02p-0317_emc-000199.txt.

24. Theresa Dale, PhD, CCN, NP, "Dr. Lendon Smith, M.D. there is an enormous population suffering from side effects associated with

aspartame, yet have no idea why drugs...,"
http://drleonardcoldwell.com/explosive-facts-about-sugar-substitutes-a-sweet-delight-or-toxic-poison/?print=print.

25. Mark Gold, "Reported Aspartame Toxicity Reactions," FDA, January 12, 2003,
http://www.fda.gov/ohrms/dockets/dailys/03/jan03/012203/02p-0317_emc-000199.txt.

Chapter 9

1. Siegel GJ, Agranoff BW, Albers RW, "Serotonin Involvement in Physiological Function and Behavior," Basic Neurochemistry: Molecular, Cellular and Medical Aspects. 6th edition. Lippincott-Raven; 1999.

2. University of Cambridge, "Serotonin levels affect the brain's response to anger," University of Cambridge, Biological Psychiatry journal, 15 Sep 2011, http://www.cam.ac.uk/research/news/serotonin-levels-affect-the-brain's-response-to-anger.

3. Molly Crockett Ph.D., "Serotonin levels affect the brain's response to anger," University of Cambridge, Biological Psychiatry journal, 15 Sep 2011, http://www.cam.ac.uk/research/news/serotonin-levels-affect-the-brain's-response-to-anger.

4. Saori C. Tanaka, Nicolas Schweighofer, Shuji Asahi, Kazuhiro Shishida, Yasumasa Okamoto, Shigeto Yamawaki, Kenji Doya, "Serotonin Differentially Regulates Short- and Long-Term Prediction of Rewards in the Ventral and Dorsal Striatum," Plos One, December 19, 2007http://dx.doi.org/10.1371/journal.pone.0001333, http://journals.plos.org/plosone/article?id=10.1371%2Fjournal.pone.0001333.

5. University of Bristol, "Brain Basics. The fundamentals of neuroscience." MRC Centre for Synaptic Plasticity, University of Bristol, School of Medical Sciences, October 5, 2011, http://www.bris.ac.uk/synaptic/basics/basics-4.html.

6. Julia Kaletka, "Chemical Messenger Research Project." Prezi, "Serotonin", Bristol University. "Serotonin", Princeton University. "Migraine Headaches", University of Maryland Medical Center. "Low serotonin-receptor levels linked to depression", Washington University at St. Louis. "What is Serotonin and What Does It Do?",

Macalester College. 20 November 2013,
https://prezi.com/6_2vlb3a7xjq/chemical-messenger-research-project/.

7. Christian P. Muller, Barry Jacobs, "Handbook of the Behavioral Neurobiology of Serotonin, Volume 21 (Handbook of Behavioral Neuroscience) 1st Edition, Academic Press; 1 edition, December 16, 2009, p 153.
8. University of Maryland, "Headaches – cluster," University of Maryland Medical Center (UMMC), http://umm.edu/health/medical/reports/articles/headaches-cluster.
9. Psych Central Staff, "Frequently Asked Questions about Serotonin," PsychCentral, 19 Feb 2008, http://psychcentral.com/lib/frequently-asked-questions-about-serotonin/.

Chapter 10

1. Brillat-Savarin. Physiologie du Goût ou, Méditations de Gastronomie Transcendante. Paris: A. Sautelet, 1826.
2. Lisa Wogan, "Jan. 22 memorial for researcher who discovered dog laughter." The Bark, January 10, 2011, http://thebark.com/content/patricia-simonet-1959-2010.
3. Dr Ad Vingerhoets, "Why Only Humans Weep," The Guardian, 15 March 2014, https://www.theguardian.com/lifeandstyle/2014/mar/15/ask-grown-up-why-we-cry-when-sad.
4. Kristin Andrews, "Hope Ferdowsian and psychologist Gay Bradshaw, have shown that captive animals do indeed suffer…" Routledge, The Animal Mind: An Introduction to the Philosophy of Animal Cognition, November 21, 2014, p 156.
5. Arin Greenwood, "What It Means To Say A Dolphin Committed Suicide." The Huffington Post, June 14, 2014, http://www.huffingtonpost.com.au/entry/dolphin-commits-suicide_n_5491513.
6. Aristotle, Eudemus; quoted by Plutarch, Consolation to Apollonius 27.
7. Justin Nobel, "Do Animals Commit Suicide? A Scientific Debate." TIME, Mar. 19, 2010,

http://content.time.com/time/health/article/0,8599,1973486,00.html
.

8. Seeker, "Animal Suicide Sheds Light on Human Behavior," Discovery Communications, Mar 10, 2010, http://www.seeker.com/animal-suicide-sheds-light-on-human-behavior-1765032181.html#news.discovery.com.

9. Suzannah Hills, "Bears kept in tiny cages by Chinese for their bile 'commit suicide'..." The Daily Mail, 4 February 2012, http://www.dailymail.co.uk/news/article-2095904/Bears-held-harvest-bile-going-hunger-strikes-way-escape-captivity.html#ixzz4Hvm9gzsO..."

10. Daisy Freund, "How Animal Welfare Leads to Better Meat: A Lesson From Spain." The Atlantic, Aug 25, 2011, http://www.theatlantic.com/health/archive/2011/08/how-animal-welfare-leads-to-better-meat-a-lesson-from-spain/244127/.

11. Neil Risch, PhD, Richard Herrell, PhD, Thomas Lehner, PhD, Kung-Yee Liang, PhD, Lindon Eaves, PhD, Josephine Hoh, PhD, Andrea Griem, BS, Maria Kovacs, PhD, Jurg Ott, PhD, Kathleen Ries Merikangas, PhD, "Interaction Between the Serotonin Transporter Gene (5-HTTLPR), Stressful Life Events, and Risk of Depression." US National Library of Medicine, National Institutes of Health, June 17, 2009, http://www.ncbi.nlm.nih.gov/pmc/articles/PMC2938776/.

12. Jonathan Savitz, Ph.D, Wayne C Drevets, M.D. "Bipolar and Major Depressive Disorder: Neuroimaging the Developmental-Degenerative Divide." US National Library of Medicine, National Institutes of Health, Apr 22, 2010, http://www.ncbi.nlm.nih.gov/pmc/articles/PMC2858318/.

13. Mufti Ebrahim Desai, "The Fiqh of Halal and Haram Animals." Darul Iftaa, Madrassah In'aamiyyah, http://www.central-mosque.com/index.php/General-Fiqh/the-fiqh-of-halal-and-haram-animals.html.

14. "Dietary Laws". Encyclopedia Judaica. Jerusalem: Keter Publishing House. 1971.

15. Islamic Halal Gulf Standards, Islamic Gulf Law Standards (GS 993/1998).

16. William H. Shea, "Clean and Unclean Meats", Biblical Research Institute". Dec, 1998.

17. Peta, "The Chicken Industry", http://www.peta.org/issues/animals-used-for-food/factory-farming/chickens/chicken-industry/.
18. Consumer Reports, "How safe is that chicken? Most tested broilers were contaminated", Consumer Reports magazine, January 2010, http://www.consumerreports.org/cro/magazine-archive/2010/january/food/chicken-safety/overview/chicken-safety-ov.htm,
19. Karen Davis, PhD, "Broilers now grow so rapidly that the heart...," United Poultry Concerns, 4 May 2015, http://www.upc-online.org/respect/150504_a_chicken_named_viva_changed_my_life.html.
20. Dr. Ben Kim. "Eating Bacon & Skinless Chicken May Cause Bladder Cancer," Dec 02, 2006, http://drbenkim.com/blog/2006/12/bacon-skinless-chicken-may-cause.html.

Chapter 11

1. The Stone Age, https://web.archive.org/web/20100818123718/http://www.nhm.ac.uk/about-us/news/2010/august/oldest-tool-use-and-meat-eating-revealed75831.html
2. The Bronze Age, "Beye, Charles Rowan", Jan 1963, "Lucretius and Progress". The Classical Journal, p 58 & p 160–169.
3. Encyclopædia Britannica, "the Iron Age," Nov, 2015, https://www.britannica.com/event/Iron-Age.
4. American Chemistry Council, "petroleum is a carbon-rich raw material," American Chemistry Council, Plastics Industry Producer Statistics Group, 2005, https://plastics.americanchemistry.com/How-Plastics-Are-Made/.
5. Carleton College, "580,000 pieces of plastic per a square kilometre...," 5. Carleton College, August 02, 2016, http://serc.carleton.edu/NAGTWorkshops/health/case_studies/plastics.html.
6. Carolyn Barry, "Plastic Breaks Down in Ocean, After All -- And Fast," National Geographic Society, August 20, 2009,

http://news.nationalgeographic.com/news/2009/08/090820-plastic-decomposes-oceans-seas.html.

7. Ecology Center, "Adverse Health Effects Of Plastics," Ecology Center Berkley California, http://ecologycenter.org/factsheets/adverse-health-effects-of-plastics/.

8. David Heath, "Meet the 'Rented White Coats' Who Defend Toxic Chemicals," Vice News, February 8, 2016, https://news.vice.com/article/meet-the-rented-white-coats-who-defend-toxic-chemicals.

9. Janet Raloff, "Bottled water may contain 'hormones': Plastics," Science News, March 12, 2009, https://www.sciencenews.org/blog/science-public/bottled-water-may-contain-'hormones'-plastics.

10. Yale Universit, "Prenatal Exposure To BPA and DES May Increase Breast Cancer Risk," Yale University, May 28, 2010, http://news.yale.edu/2010/05/28/prenatal-exposure-bpa-and-des-may-increase-breast-cancer-risk.

11. Hannah Nichols, Dr. Helen Webberley, "Estrogen: How Does Estrogen Work?" 1 April 2016, http://www.medicalnewstoday.com/articles/277177.php.

12. FDA, "Breast Cancer—Men Get It Too." U.S. Food and Drug Administration FDA, June 27, 2014, http://www.fda.gov/ForConsumers/ConsumerUpdates/ucm402937.htm.

13. Pratap Kumar, Navneet Magon, "Hormones in pregnancy." US National Library of Medicine National Institutes of Health, 2012 Oct-Dec; 53(4): 179–183. http://www.ncbi.nlm.nih.gov/pmc/articles/PMC3640235/.

14. Dr. Ronald Hoffman, "Estrogen dominance syndrome." October 4, 2013, http://drhoffman.com/article/estrogen-dominance-syndrome-2/.

15. Cheryl S. Watson, Yow-Juin Jeng, Jutatip Guptarak, "Endocrine disruption via estrogen receptors that participate in nongenomic signaling pathways." US National Library of Medicine National Institutes of Health, Feb 12, 2011, http://www.ncbi.nlm.nih.gov/pmc/articles/PMC3106143/.

16. Brad J. King, MS, MFS, "Counterfeit Estrogens and Your Metabolism." Alive Australia, Apr 24, 2015, http://www.alive.com/health/counterfeit-estrogens-and-your-metabolism/.

17. Stanford Report, "5 Questions: Feldman on risk of bisphenol A in plastic bottles." Stanford University, April 30, 2008, http://news.stanford.edu/news/2008/april30/med-5qbpa-043008.html.

18. Harvey PW, Darbre P., "Endocrine disrupters and human health: could oestrogenic chemicals in body care cosmetics," US National Library of Medicine National Institutes of Health, May-Jun. 2004, 24(3):167-76. http://www.ncbi.nlm.nih.gov/pubmed/15211609.

Chapter 12

1. U.S. National Library of Medicine, "How many chromosomes do people have?" U.S. National Library of Medicine, August 23, 2016, https://ghr.nlm.nih.gov/primer/basics/howmanychromosomes.

2. Katherine Harmon, "weight gain in social circles," Scientific American, May 5, 2011, http://www.scientificamerican.com/article/social-spread-obesity/.

3. Tagtow A, Robien K, Bergquist E, Bruening M, Dierks L, Hartman BE, Robinson-O'Brien R, Steinitz T, Tahsin B, Underwood T, Wilkins J. "people have a natural wish to conform to the standards of a group…" American Journal of the Academy of Nutrition and Dietetics, US National Library of Medicine National Institutes of Health, March, 2014, http://www.ncbi.nlm.nih.gov/pubmed/24534371.

4. Alex Caldon, ""If you tell a lie big enough and keep repeating it…," Easterly Press, The Quest for Truth, 2007, p 165.

5. Hilmar Hoffmann, John Broadwin, Volker R. Berghahn, "The most brilliant propagandist technique will yield…,", Berghahn Books, The Triumph of Propaganda: Film and National Socialism, 1933-1945 v1, August 30, 1997, p 140.

6. George Carlin, "It's a big club and you ain't in it…," Shelf-Life Productions LLC, Alternative Reel, Top 10 George Carlin Quotes, http://www.alternativereel.com/soc/display_article.php?id=0000000 019.

Suggestions

1. Desiderius Erasmus, "Prevention is better than cure." Brainy Quote, http://www.brainyquote.com/quotes/keywords/prevention.html.
2. Benjamin Franklin, "An ounce of prevention is worth a pound of cure." Good Reads, http://www.goodreads.com/quotes/247269-an-ounce-of-prevention-is-worth-a-pound-of-cure.
3. Karen E. Haneke, M.S., Bonnie L. Carson, M.S.," Review of Toxicological Literature." National Institute of Environmental Health Sciences, Oct 2001, https://ntp.niehs.nih.gov/ntp/htdocs/chem_background/exsumpdf/fluorosilicates_508.pdf.
4. William Hirzy, "fluoride that otherwise would be an air and water…" Dan Fagin, Scientific American, Jan 2008, http://www.scientificamerican.com/article/second-thoughts-on-fluoride/?responsive=false.
5. American Dental Association ADA, "old "should consider using water that has no or low levels of fluoride" Fluoridation facts, ADA Statement Commemorating the 60th Anniversary of Community Water Fluoridation, American Dental Association at 1-312-440-2879., http://www.ada.org/~/media/ADA/Member%20Center/FIles/fluoridation_facts.ashx.
6. World Health Organization Collaborating Centre for Education, Training, and Research in Oral Health, Malmö University, Sweden, March 30, 2013, http://www.mah.se/CAPP/.
7. Dr. Doull, ""[W]e've gone with the status quo regarding fluoride for many years—for too long," Scientific American,, Jan 2008, www.fluoridealert.org/researchers/nrc/panelists/.
8. National Research Council, "Fluoride in drinking water" a scientific review of EPA's standards. National Academies Press, Washington D.C, 2008, www.nap.edu/catalog.php?record_id=11571.
9. Excerpts of NAS's findings, www.fluoridealert.org/researchers/nrc/findings/.
10. Excerpts of NAS's recommendations, www.fluoridealert.org/researchers/nrc/recommendations/
11. FDA's letters confirming this disapproval of fluoride in supplements, see: www.fluoridealert.org/researchers/fda/not-approved/

12. The two fluoride supplements that FDA has rejected are Enziflur (a fluoride/vitamin combination) and prenatal fluoride supplements. See: www.fluoridealert.org/uploads/enziflur-1975.pdf and www.fluoridealert.org/articles/fda-1966/.

13. For an extensive compilation of quotes from dental researchers discussing this consensus, see: www.fluoridealert.org/studies/caries04/.

14. According to the CDC, "fluoride prevents dental caries predominately after eruption of the tooth into the mouth, and its actions primarily are topical for both adults and children." Centers for Disease Control (1999). Morbidity and Mortality Weekly Report 48: 933-40.

15. Yu Y, et al. (1996). Neurotransmitter and receptor changes in the brains of fetuses from areas of endemic fluorosis. Chinese Journal of Endemiology 15:257-259; re-published in Fluroide 2008, 41(2):134–138.

16. Dr. Melinda Ratini, "A pH level measures how acid or alkaline something is…," WebMD, Sonya Collins, Reviewed by Michael Dansinger, MD on March 11, 2016, http://www.webmd.com/diet/a-z/alkaline-diets.

17. Dr. Margaret Cuomo, "More than 40 years after Nixon launched the war on cancer…," Tom Blackwell, National Post, March 15, 2013, http://news.nationalpost.com/news/war-on-cancer.

18. President Richard M. Nixon, "an extensive campaign to find a cure for cancer." The American Presidency Project, January 22, 1971, http://www.presidency.ucsb.edu/ws/?pid=3110.

19. President Barack Obama, "Our recovery plan will invest in electronic health records…," Jenna Adamson, USA Today, January 14, 2016, http://www.usatoday.com/story/opinion/2016/01/14/obama-state-union-address-biden-cure-cancer-column/78753580/.

20. Health Impact News, "Since the war on cancer began on 1971, more than 14,800,000…," Health Impact News, August 15, 2014, http://healthimpactnews.com/2014/the-cancer-industry-is-too-prosperous-to-allow-a-cure/.

21. Drug Watch, "Big Pharma," https://www.drugwatch.com/manufacturer/.

22. Larry D. Sasich, PharmD, MPH, FASHP, "This starts out in the first year of medical school..." Media Education Foundation, 2006, http://www.mediaed.org/transcripts/Big-Bucks-BIg-Pharma-Transcript.pdf.
23. Gene Carbona, "No matter where you spend money," Media Education Foundation, 2006, http://www.mediaed.org/transcripts/Big-Bucks-BIg-Pharma-Transcript.pdf.
24. Kelly D. Brownell, M. R. C. Greenwood, Eliot Stellar, E. Eileen Shrager, "Yo-Yo Diet," 1986, Physiology &Behaviour, Vol. 38, pp. 459—464.
25. Sylvia P. Onusic, PhD, CNS, LDN, "Violent Behavior: A Solution in Plain Sight." The Weston A. Price Foundation, April 22, 2013, http://www.westonaprice.org/uncategorized/violent-behavior-a-solution-in-plain-sight/
26. William Kraus, M.D., associate professor, medicine, Duke University Medical Center, Durham, N.C.; Richard A. Stein, M.D., professor, clinical medicine, Weill Cornell Medical Center, New York City; Nov. 7, 2002, The New England Journal of Medicine.

Quotes Citations

- Frank Zappa, "A mind is like a parachute. It doesn't work if it is not open." Good Reads, http://www.goodreads.com/quotes/33052-a-mind-is-like-a-parachute-it-doesn-t-work-if.
- Adam Musselli, "Ignorance is not a bliss nor it will ever be and knowledge is not power until it's applied" The MindTech Institute, The Day We Gave Up Health, p 5, http://www.TheMindTechInstitute.com.
- Marie Curie, ""Nothing in life is to be feared...," Brainy Quotes, http://www.brainyquote.com/quotes/quotes/m/mariecurie389010.html
- Adam Musselli, "In order to understand something you first need to liberate yourself from it." The MindTech Institute, The Day We Gave Up Health, p 6, http://www.TheMindTechInstitute.com.
- Martin Niemöller, "First they came for the Socialists...," Holocaust Encyclopedia, https://www.ushmm.org/wlc/en/article.php?ModuleId=10007392.

- George Orwell, "In times of universal deceit…," Unsigned, written by Antonio Gramsci in collaboration with Palmiro Togliatti, L'Ordine Nuovo, 21 June 1919, Vol. 1, No. 7.
- Adam Musselli, "It is not a disgrace to be deceived;" The MindTech Institute, The Day We Gave Up Health, p 13, http://www.TheMindTechInstitute.com.
- Nelson Mandela, "Education is the most powerful weapon…," The United Nations, http://www.un.org/en/globalissues/briefingpapers/efa/quotes.shtml.
- Adam Musselli, "Ignorance is not a bliss nor it will ever be…," The MindTech Institute, The Day We Gave Up Health, p 16, http://www.TheMindTechInstitute.com.
- Michael Pollan "What an extraordinary achievement for a civilization…," Good Reads, http://www.goodreads.com/quotes/224525-what-an-extraordinary-achievement-for-a-civilization-to-have-developed.
- Karl Pilkington, "With evolution, things are always changing, so I sort of think…," QuoteCourt, http://quotecourt.com/karl-pilkington-quote-313893.
- Jordan Maxwell, "Always trust someone who is seeking the truth …," Jordan Maxwell Show, https://jordanmaxwellshow.com/blog/tag/astrology/.
- Adam Musselli, "There are lots of half –truths around…," The MindTech Institute, The Day We Gave Up Health, p 24, http://www.TheMindTechInstitute.com.
- Tupac Shakur, "Don't believe everything you hear…," Good Reads, http://www.goodreads.com/quotes/865859-don-t-believe-everything-you-hear-real-eyes-realize-real-lies.
- Lord Alfred Tennyson, "A lie is half-truth is the darkest of all lies" The Grandmother, The Literature Network, http://www.online-literature.com/tennyson/4087/.
- David Suzuki, "Any politician or scientist who tells you these…," AzQuotes, http://www.azquotes.com/quote/1432286.
- Adam Musselli, "I always wonder, how we can eat something…," The MindTech Institute, The Day We Gave Up Health, p 45, http://www.TheMindTechInstitute.com.

- Sean Covey, "we become what we repeatedly do." Good Reads, http://www.goodreads.com/quotes/272578-we-become-what-we-repeatedly-do.
- Warren Buffett, "The chains of habit are too light to be felt…," Brainy Quotes, http://www.brainyquote.com/quotes/quotes/w/warrenbuff384858.html.
- Unknown, "You are what you eat so don't be fast, cheap, easy or fake." Jar Of Quotes, http://www.jarofquotes.com/view.php?id=you-are-what-you-eat-so-dont-be-fast-cheap-easy-or-fake.
- Jeanette Jenkins, "Every living cell in your body is made from the food you eat…," Move Me Quotes, http://www.movemequotes.com/14603/11508_753445198005137_186449078_n/.
- Oprah Winfrey "My drug of choice is food. I use food for the same reasons an addict uses drugs…,"Donna Duggan, My Body And soul, December 4, 2010, http://www.bodyandsoul.com.au/diet/lose-weight/oprahs-battle-with-weight-loss/news-story/2857e0db6135ea2c9aabc67b8669e971.
- Deepak Chopra, M.D, "Being addicted to food brings suffering…,"What Are You Hungry For?: The Chopra Solution to Permanent Weight Loss, Well-Being, and Lightness of Soul, Harmony; 1 edition, Nov 12, 2013, p 10.
- Jamie Oliver, "Homicide is 0.8% of deaths. Diet-related disease is over 60%…," AzQuotes, http://www.azquotes.com/quote/850940.
- James St. James, "I give you bitter pills, in a sugar coating…," Good reads, http://www.goodreads.com/quotes/168558-i-give-you-bitter-pills-in-a-sugar-coating-the.
- Urban Dictionary, (hang-gree) hangry:adj. A state of anger caused by a lack of food…," http://www.urbandictionary.com/define.php?term=Hangry.
- H.G. Wells, "Hunger and a lack of blood-corpuscles take all the manhood from a man." Good Reads, http://www.goodreads.com/quotes/333819-hunger-and-a-lack-of-blood-corpuscles-take-all-the-manhood.

- Mahatma Gandhi, "The greatness of a nation can be judged by the way...," Good Reads, http://www.goodreads.com/quotes/340-the-greatness-of-a-nation-and-its-moral-progress-can.
- Immanuel Kant, "He who is cruel to animals becomes hard also in his...," Brainy Quotes, http://www.brainyquote.com/quotes/quotes/i/immanuelka390204.html.
- Rev. Dr. Martin Luther King, Jr., "The time is always right to do what is right." Oberlin College Archives, http://www.oberlin.edu/external/EOG/BlackHistoryMonth/MLK/MLK mainpage.html.
- Mahatma Gandhi, "Earth provides enough to satisfy every man's needs...," Good Reads, http://www.goodreads.com/quotes/30431-earth-provides-enough-to-satisfy-every-man-s-needs-but-not.
- Prof. Guy McPherson, "If you really think the environment is less important than the economy...," Oleg Komlik, Economic Sociology and Political Economy, August 20, 2014, https://economicsociology.org/2014/08/20/if-you-think-the-economy-is-more-important-than-the-environment-try-holding-your-breath-while-counting-your-money/.
- Malcolm X, "If you're not careful, the newspapers will have you hating the people...," Good Reads, http://www.goodreads.com/quotes/280633-if-you-re-not-careful-the-newspapers-will-have-you-hating.
- Mark Twain, "It's easier to fool people than to convince them they have been fooled." The Quotepedia, http://www.thequotepedia.com/its-easier-to-fool-people-than-to-convince-them-they-have-been-fooled-mark-twain/.
- Jacque Fresco, "Democracy is a con game. It's a word invented to placate people to make them accept a given institution...," Good Reads, http://www.goodreads.com/quotes/725613-democracy-is-a-con-game-it-s-a-word-invented-to.
- Albert Einstein, "The world is a dangerous place to live; not because...," Prof. Daniel Palanker, Stanford University, http://web.stanford.edu/~palanker/wisdom.html.

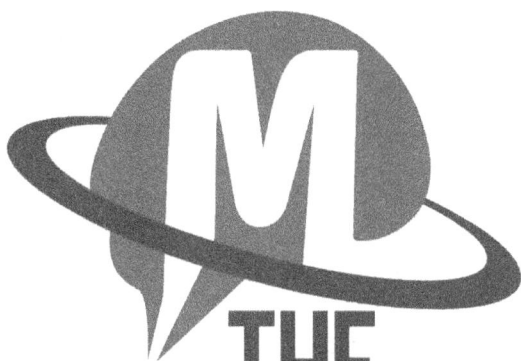

THE
MINDTECH
INSTITUTE

www.themindtechinstitute.com
www.mti.edu.au

The MindTech Institute

Offers a range of online courses

Now you can study any of our courses online and get fully qualified by simply enrolling online and enjoy studying at your own pace using our easy and user-friendly online learning system.
www.themindtechinstitute.com OR www.mti.edu.au

All our diplomas and advanced diplomas are fully accredited and recognized worldwide. The MindTech Institute is a Registered Training Organization (RTO No. 41585).

Advanced Diploma (Associate Degree) of Leadership & Management BSB61015

Diploma (Associate Degree) of Counselling CHC51015

Neuro-Linguistic Programming Training (NLP) Practitioner

Neuro-Linguistic Programming Training (NLP) Master Practitioner

Hypnosis (Hypnotherapy) Training Practitioner

Hypnosis (Hypnotherapy) Training Master Practitioner

Life Management Training (Life Coaching)

Advanced Sales Training

Customer Service Training – Handling Customers

Time Management Training

Advanced Presentation Training

Leadership Training Program

Emotional Intelligence EQ Training

Stress Management Training

Personal Effectiveness Training

The MindTech Institute

Fast-Track And Recognition of Prior Learning (RPL)

You can also take advantage of our Fast-Track and Recognition of Prior Learning RPL programs and obtain an Advanced Diploma (Associate Degree) in less time - *conditions apply*…

All information are available at The MindTech Institute's website www.themindtechinstitute.com OR www.mti.edu.au

Various Advanced Diplomas and Diplomas (Associate Degrees) are available through our RPL and Fast-Track accelerated programs:

Advanced Diploma of Marketing and Communication BSB61315

Advanced Diploma of Leadership & Management BSB61015

Diploma of Hospitality Management SIT50416

Diploma of Counselling CHC51015

Check out www.themindtechinstitute.com Or www.mti.edu.au for more…

BEAUTY IN CHAOS

An Inner Journey to Restoring Love, Hope, and Freedom

By Denise Sivilay

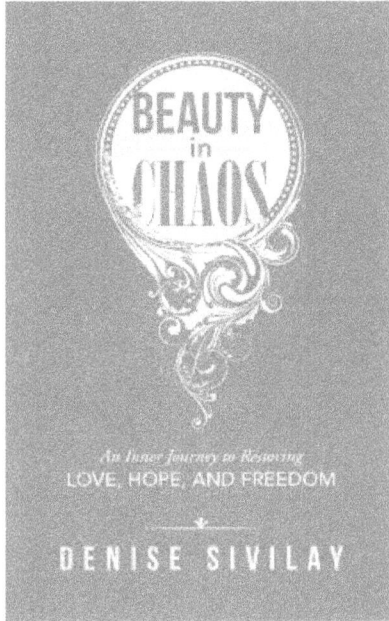

In her late twenties, Denise Sivilay began seeking ways to heal her life and purge herself of addictions and an attachment to a mind-set that had corrupted her emotionally, mentally, physically, and spiritually.

In Beauty in Chaos, Sivilay shares the life-changing lessons about love and life she has gleaned along the path of seeking self-love, healing, forgiveness, and true happiness. She narrates the stories of her life: from her birth in Laos in 1980, to escaping that violent environment and moving to Australia at three years old, to growing up without a father figure, to being a victim of her own self-sabotaging patterns and limiting beliefs.

From the good to the bad, Beauty in Chaos presents a journey where every event plays a role in the story. Sivilay shares how she was able to find happiness in the midst of sadness, and she encourages you to see the beauty in yourself, discover your own worth, and learn the value of real joy and love.

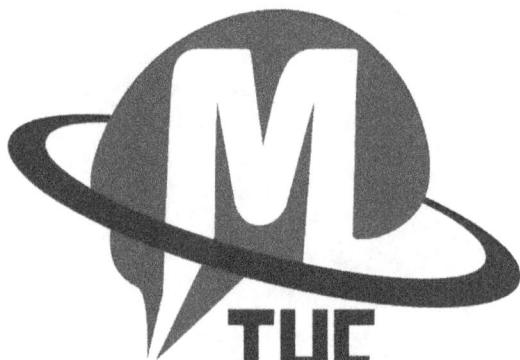

THE MINDTECH INSTITUTE

www.themindtechinstitute.com
www.mti.edu.au

THE MINDTECH INSTITUTE

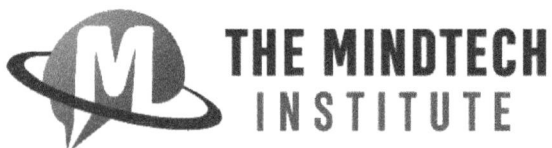

Email: info@themindtechinstitute.com

Websites: www.themindtechinstitute.com

www.mti.edu.au

www.ingramcontent.com/pod-product-compliance
Lightning Source LLC
Chambersburg PA
CBHW021852020426
42334CB00013B/303